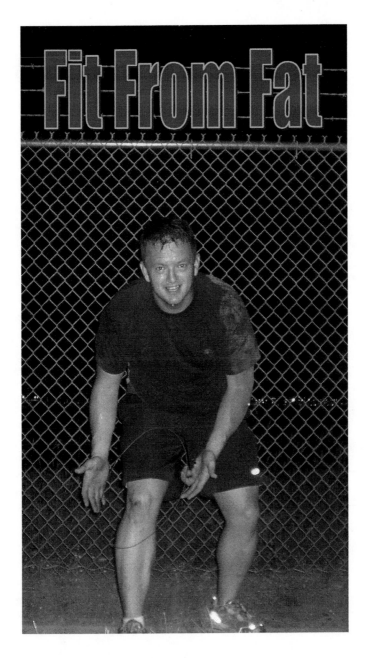

Fit From Fat

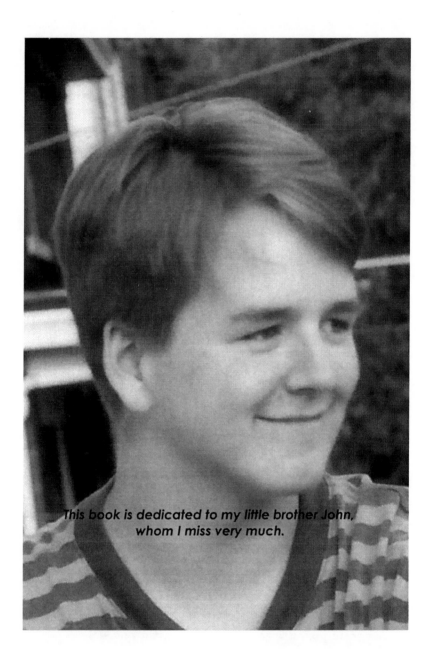

This book is dedicated to my little brother John, whom I miss very much.

Table of Contents

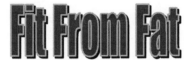

My story is not special.

What do I mean? Surely there are some who have opened this book that would find it special to go from being obese to becoming a fit person without surgery, without medicine. What I mean is that I believe that anyone, ANYONE at all can make the same decisions I did and change their life. There are different degrees to which some of us may be genetically advantaged to achieve certain things, but anyone can change their circumstance for the better if they find themselves yearning for change.

There is no time at which it is too late to start, save the closing of your casket, and there is no positive change in your life too trivial to pursue. It comes down to what you want for yourself.

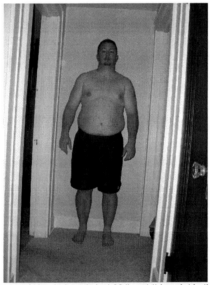

285 lbs, and I had already lost 30 lbs at this point in time. I did not take any 315 lb. pictures, though now I wish I had.

Chapter 1 - Background

0-32

I led an active childhood full of wandering the neighborhood I lived in....
bike rides amongst friends.... swimming whenever we could get to a pool.
I never had a particularly strong interest in sports when I was younger. I
ran a 4-mile race when I was about 10 years old and puked at the end of
it.

As I entered high school I participated in some sports but never had the
spark or natural talent to make any varsity starting teams. I tried football
my freshman and sophomore years, but lacked the athleticism or
aggressiveness to do much on the gridiron.

I ran track, just because, and I ran in the two mile after realizing I would
never be fast enough to do sprints. I also tried my hand at throwing the
discus. I joined the diving team and even made good progress until I was
able to do a 2 ½ reverse, up until I under-rotated twice in one practice
smacking hard on my back, and promptly walked over to the lap lanes
and asked to be put on the swimming team. I participated but never led
any events.

When I moved to a new high school my junior year, I played on the golf
team and enjoyed that a lot more than football, but again, never did
much to distinguish myself there.

With my senior year coming to a close I was of average fitness with
nothing to physically distinguish myself, but knowing that college was
coming, and I wanted to meet cute girls, I set out during the summer to
change my outline. I figured I could run, so I started doing that. I ran the
first day something like ½ mile. The next day 1 mile.... and so on...until by
the end of the summer, I was running some runs in the range of 9 miles
and feeling very good about that. I was slender, full of energy and ready
to go to college!

As I entered collegiate life at the University of Cincinnati I kept up my
running and even met a good friend to run with on a regular basis. I
would run loops around campus, and I would run on the track when
weather was inclement. I listened to music on a Walkman cassette player
and steadily got faster. It is in my nature when exercising to gradually
push myself to do more by either going faster or going farther. The best

speed run I can recall was a day that I decided to do 10 miles on the outdoor track (40 laps) and see how fast I could complete it. I ended up running 10 miles in 57:45, which, at fewer than 6 minutes per mile average, blows my mind now, 15 years later. The longest run I remember from those days was in the range of 19 miles or so, running with my friend Jason, when we were training for the Blue Ash marathon, which I never ended up running. He did, and ran very well.

As the first year of college wound down, I ran less and played basketball more and more. I really enjoyed basketball and the atmosphere at UC at the time was very much a basketball friendly place. I even enjoyed many games playing on the court with the varsity players from the team during the off-season.

Towards the end of my first year of school there, it became apparent that my chosen major of Mechanical Engineering held no sway over my heart and I needed to find a flight school to become a pilot (my current profession as I write this.) I dropped out of school and before entering flight school at the Kent State University; I joined the National Guard to help defray the costs of flight lessons, and went through basic and advanced training for the Army at Fort Knox in Kentucky. I became much stronger in the upper body during those training months, and still held enough of my earlier running skills to be the fastest in my unit at the two mile run for all of basic training, and the first few years of service afterwards.

I never kept up with my fitness though and only ran when I had to for physical fitness tests, and played basketball for fun, but never pursued a serious fitness regimen. I ate the way I had been able to eat when I was 19 and running all the time. I basically ate whatever I felt like with no concern to quantity or quality of what I was putting in my body. Through college, it was very common for me to order a large pizza and a two liter of soda and eat it all myself. I always had several sandwiches when eating at the cafeteria, not just one. Most meals always included a soft drink, a full meal, and a dessert. It just seemed that was the way it was, I didn't think about it much. I thought of myself as reasonably fit and didn't really look at who I was truly becoming.

Pounds become tens of pounds, and where I had weighed as low as 160 during my freshman year (TOO light for me) I was up in the range of 230 by the time I was graduating from Kent State 5 and a half years later, but still figured I was "OK."

Now I leave school and transition to developing a career. Every year from age 23 on I would add 5-15 lbs, and I gradually started to realize that I was becoming "big Mike" as the years went by. I went from wearing a size 34 pants in early college, on up to size 44 by the time I was 32 years old. I went from large shirts to XXL shirts and those were even kind of tight depending on who made them. I had ballooned over time, and the gradual pace at which life puts it on, had allowed me the silly self-indulgence of making excuses all along the way, and not taking control of who I was becoming.

At the age of 32, I would order two large pizzas for the family, and I would eat one of them, and my wife and kids would split the other. I would cycle from snack cake to snack cake, eating whatever suited me that week....hohos, little debbies, boston cream pies....you name it.

I would buy a bag of jellybeans and it would disappear in one sitting in front of the computer, surfing the internet. I would buy candy bars in bunches. I would drink soda in large quantities.

Sure, there were times when I found a little motivation and tried drinking diet soda for a while, or eating better. I would exercise for a few days. No commitment. No burning flame that could not be extinguished, making change in my life.

32 and on...

Then during the week of March 10th, 2006 a lot of motivating factors all occurred within one short time to light my fuse.

I really started to feel bad about how I was looking and feeling, and the way it impacted the life I was leading as a father to my daughters. No one said anything, but I was starting to take a hard look at who and what I was as a person. I sat in my large bathtub in my house and looked at the fat that had accumulated on my body, and the fact that I had finally achieved the infamous "cankles" where the calves and ankles combine with no discernible break giving one the "fat" look at the feet. That smacked me upside the head hard when I saw that.

I read some information about a coworker of mine, Tyler Darby, who had taken his life back after fighting off testicular cancer and changed his shape and lifestyle from overweight and going the wrong way, to fit and going the right way. He trained for triathlons with a passion and documented his achievements on a website for all to see. From his website I linked to and found a story about Dick and Rick Hoyt, a father and son team who compete in triathlons and marathons together, even though the son has cerebral palsy and can only move his head since birth. A son who the doctors had encouraged the father to "let go" and the father never gave up and found out Rick's passion was sports and he wanted to join in, so they started running races together with Dick pushing him in a wheelchair. They went on to run marathons, and compete in triathlons with Dick riding a bike equipped for both of them, and towing Rick behind in a life raft for the swim portions of triathlons.

Prior to discovering Rick's passions, Dick had never been an athlete of any kind and in his 40's he started running, and learned to swim so he could participate with his son. Reading their website and stories brought me to tears at the sheer humanity of two people devoting themselves to each other like these two had. Dick and Rick are still my heroes in the athletic realm. Their story was found in detail on the website they had at www.teamhoyt.com.

The fire was lit that week, and I promised myself to keep it fueled from this point forward. I started walking every night and incorporating some exercise in every single day. I researched on the internet about counting calories and how to eat to lose weight. I came to understand after reading a book called "Burn the Fat, Feed the Muscle" that I wanted to lose **fat** and not *weight*. I learned eating strategies and goal setting strategies to get me where I wanted to go.

I used Slim Fast shakes for about 6 weeks to get a handle on how many calories I was actually eating compared to what I needed. I learned that I could only deficit my calorie needs by about 15-17% below what I needed just to maintain weight if I wanted to lose fat effectively. I had determined from formulas found online and in the book I mentioned that at my starting weight, I required around 2450 calories just to maintain my weight. This "maintenance" calorie load would drop as I lost weight too. So each day, early on, I was trying to take in between 2000 and 2100 calories. This worked for me.

I made weight goals at first for 90-day periods that were based upon a reasonable weight loss of 2-3 lbs per week. These were written on a fluorescent index card in permanent marker and kept in my wallet on top of everything else, so every time I opened my wallet I was reminded of what I was going for.

I would walk until my feet were sore, listening to the radio. I often walked in the evening after my daughters had gone to sleep so I could not take that time away from them. This was in a large way something I thought of as giving back to them. I would try to give them more years with their father, more fun with their father as I would do more being fit, and most of all setting a good example of living a balanced life. I decided that I could live with my girls growing up overweight, because I was not a bad person when I was obese, in fact, I am not better a person now that I am in shape. What I could not live with was if I set the bad example of being obese myself and felt like they grew up overweight and were hurt by watching that in me.

At night, walking the sidewalks of my town, I would see the same cop car go by again and again, and often wondered what they thought of this guy out there walking for hours on end in the night.

"I don't live to eat, I eat to live."

Now, I don't know who might have been the first to say this, but I know I heard it from my mother as I started to visibly show my progress, and she told me where she heard it. It seems that my grandfather had a heart condition (which eventually took him 3 months before I was born) and he was under fairly strict orders from his doctor for a good portion of his adult life about what he could eat. My grandmother would lament the fact that he could not join the family in the desserts she prepared and he would say, "Mary, I don't live to eat, I eat to live."

For a long portion of my initial weight loss this became my mantra when I would think about controlling my diet and making new habits. I came to remind myself of this phrase to keep the concept at the front of my consciousness that food is just fuel. It is not the marrow of my life, but simply the fuel that allows me to enjoy the laughter of my children, the beauty of a sunset and so on.

As my progress started to become markedly obvious I started receiving all kinds of positive reinforcement from everyone who knew me. My family, my coworkers, people of my community would all heap on the compliments and smiles and happy moments that came to me a major reward for what I had done so far. My time on my feet gave me the opportunity to reflect that I could not allow this to become a major driving factor in my efforts for several reasons.

The first is that this praise was sure to be temporary in nature. Eventually, the image of Mike as a fat guy would dissipate in folk's memory banks and they wouldn't be shocked to see a slim me, and would no longer comment. I understood this. It would happen to me too. After a period of conditioning we all take most everything for granted in our daily lives. It is human. So if the praise were a driving force, it would soon enough dwindle in magnitude and frequency and I would tend to go back to being who I didn't want to be.

Along with this, I determined that this obviously had to be something that was being done for myself and not others. Sure, it helped to drive me that I was doing better for my family, but in the end, it had to be personal. I couldn't be doing it because others approved. I couldn't listen to everyone who had advice about how their "friend" or whoever lost their weight. I had to find my path, for my reason, and have faith in myself, for myself. These reasons go along with something I would come to realize about athletic achievements later on in my progress....

Chapter 2 – Let's Get Moving!

Why did you start running?

I have no idea. Well, really, I know that I always liked running from my younger days. But the actual day I started running again during my weight loss, it hit me out of nowhere. I was walking the 6 miles I would do in a local metro park and had about one mile left to go, when the urge to run a little just popped up. I picked a tree some 50-60 yards ahead of me, and ran/jogged to it. At this time, I probably still weighed 275-280 lbs. I was totally out of breath when I went this short distance, but also exhilarated by the effort and I did 2-3 more little jogging spurts before finishing that night. The next day in the same park, I determined to go a little further (little did I know how exaggerated this process of going farther would get....). This evening I ran maybe 100-200 yards at a stretch and felt the same happiness for having done something with myself.

By the end of this week, I knew that if I pushed myself I could keep jogging for around a mile. I would find out as I went back out to work and used the treadmills in the hotel at night. My job had me flying one week on the road, and one week at home rotating. This was now early summer and I kept up the habit of running some and walking some alternatively until I did over a mile, and then two without stopping. My friend and coworker Tyler encouraged me to try to run a 5k race, and in August I signed up for one in Independence, OH. I didn't want to feel like I let myself down so I tested myself several times on the treadmills to make sure I could go that far without stopping. I did.

August 4th came and I toed the line for my first race that I could remember since high school track meets. I was nervous. Could I make it? Would I look silly? Prior to the race, my college roommate Jeff from Kent State called out my name (well my college nickname) and I was surprised to see him there. He was not running the race, but using the nearby pool with his wife and daughter and saw me. He remarked about how good I was looking and that just made my day. Jeff was always a natural athlete in college along with his younger brother. He was my favorite person to play intramural basketball with.

So the race begins. I am wearing almost brand new Nike shoes in white and orange and matching shorts and shirt. I go out with the crowd trying not to get caught up in the moment and go too fast for me. There is always a rush of excitement at these races and it is SO hard not to go too fast early on. Well, I did fine and when I hit the first mile I was blown away to hear a split time of 8:16. This was much too fast for me I thought, so I tried to force myself to slow down. I felt like it was working. I encountered the one aid station in this race where they were handing out water and found out how hard it is to drink a cup of water while running. Many races later, friends would tell me the trick of folding the cup to make it easier to drink.... I knew the second mile mark would be coming as we had turned and were headed back through the streets towards the start/finish line and was blown away when I got a 2 mile split of 16:31.

Experience told me this was WAY too fast for me, but I had also heard of race day magic and just vowed to do my best to keep going. I was huffing. I was puffing. When I came within sight of the finish line, I was really suffering and hit a point where I just couldn't take it, and I walked a short stretch to recover some. I was so devastated at this. I ran again as soon as I could, and again in a little while had to walk 50 feet or so. Then, I gathered up what I had and ran to the finish.

Wow, I was saddened, I was pissed. And revelation strikes. Who cares? I ran the race in a faster total time than I had hoped, even with the walking.... and it was my first race! I did it. I had the courage to be there. I had the drive to care. I knew I would do more and that is how I win! The low emotions faded away and I allowed myself to be proud of what I did do, instead of bummed at what I missed out on by having to walk a touch.

5k becomes 5 miles becomes a half marathon becomes...

Well, I now knew that I liked going to the races and all the fun with them. I soon found a 5-mile race on labor day that I could run close to my home. I signed up and went to the race with no idea how fast I could go for 5 straight miles, but now knew that I could just run it and have fun!

We started off and once again I was running probably a little too fast for me in the excitement of the start. After about a mile and half of running, a beautiful young lady passed me and I decided the scenery would be much better if I just sped up a bit and stayed behind her. This worked for about the next two miles and was my first introduction to the idea of what a future running friend of mine would call "butt beacons." The idea of finding a person attractive enough to pull you along at a faster clip than you would otherwise run if left to one's own willpower. It works.

After the two miles though, I just couldn't keep her pace and reverted to my little trick of walking for a short bit until I could run again. I thought this would really kill my day in terms of finishing time, but was already over that monster so I enjoyed myself. Well, now when I come back to the road that I know is near the finish line, I am astounded at how quick I have gotten this far. I mentally calculate that if I push myself a touch, I may be able to finish this 5 miles in less than 40 minutes, which would really be something for me. So I crank it up a bit, and as my eyes start to register the finish line clock I can see that it will be very close if I sprint it in...and then, she comes out of my peripheral vision! My 4 year old and 9 year old daughters have positioned themselves a few hundred yards prior to the finish line and the 4 year old decides impromptu to run it in with Daddy.

Decisions can be made in a microsecond, I know. I slowed down and took her hand and ran it in with her. 40:08. The best 8 seconds of the year if you ask me! It was funny afterwards when I realized the charity for this race was for children and she did this. I figured most people must have assumed I staged that.

So now Tyler is encouraging me to try a longer distances, to think of a half marathon. Well, I had pushed myself to run the whole 6-mile path in my favorite metro park. I thought it was possible for me, and I decided that if I could prove it again on the treadmill for 13.1 miles, I would sign up for the Towpath Half Marathon on October 8. Well, a few weeks ahead, I did the treadmill proving and got myself signed up.

Now I am learning more about distance running. This will be the longest race I have ever participated in to this point, and I learn about using energy gels from Tyler to fuel me during the run. They are essentially sugary goo designed to keep up your blood glycogen levels during endurance exercise. In fact, one of the major brands is called GU.

I had run another 5k race in September after which I used a coupon to buy a pair of shoes from the North Face called the Arnuva BOA 50 which has a cable and ratchet system instead of laces....I love them! At some point in this I learn about a guy named Dean Karnazes. He has a book out called "Ultramarathon Man" and among his many claims to fame are running 350 miles non stop (over something like 88 hours) and running in and even winning many 100 mile trail races. His story and enthusiasm catch my mind.

By now, on Tyler's urging I was keeping a blog at www.fitfromfat.blogspot.com. I will draw upon many posts from my blog and place them here to reflect the emotions I was feeling at the time of the events, rather than to try to write all new reports of my adventures. My blog post from the half marathon:

Towpath Marathon

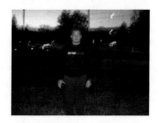

I got up this morning at about 0555 am to get a quick shower and get ready to run my first ever half marathon. The leaves are changing in Ohio now, and the temps are dropping. I was registered to run in the Towpath Marathon half marathon event today October 8, 2006. My goal in the event was first, to finish, but also to break two hours, and preferably to break a time of 1:58:11, which is the time that my good friend Tyler just completed the NYC Grete's Gallop half marathon in Central Park. Side note: I REALLY wish I could have run that with him.

I arrived at the parking lot for the event at 0700 am, just before sunrise and had to go find pins for my race bib, #1142. This was also to be my first event run with a timing chip, which is a little radio chip inside a plastic shell that is normally attached to one of your shoelaces, and registers your time at the start and finish as well as some points on the racecourse usually. I had to wear mine around my leg with a Velcro strap because the new shoes I was running in

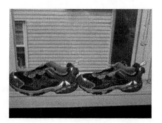

(The North Face Arnuva 50 with the BOA lacing system - see photo) do not have traditional shoelaces. It is a little steel cable that is adjusted with a dial to loosen and tighten the fit of the shoe. Absolute techno geek awesomeness! Is awesomeness a word? It is for me now. I was a little concerned about these shoes for this race, and also for a later adventure (see end of post...) but they performed very well. For running my first half marathon, I did not get any blisters or problems of any sort. I did not even have to adjust the fit of them during the race.

After securing the pins to attach my race bib to my shirt, I retreated to the warmth of our waiting Honda Civic to wait till much closer to "go time" before returning to the chill morning air. When I check the temps before leaving the house, it was showing 47 degrees.... but the sky was totally clear with a full moon hanging on overnight. I got back out of the car at about 0740 to walk down to the start line.... Of course, I had to pee one last time, and there was a mammoth line for the potties. I got in line, and when I finally got into a port o potty to go, the race starter was announcing 40 seconds till race start. No problem, I was in and out and relieved, and at the back of the line before they started. Since this race utilized timing chips, it didn't matter at all, where I started in the pack, other than starting at the back of the race means I had to maneuver around a lot of slower traffic before settling in with folks running my pace.

I crossed the starting line something like one minute behind the front of the pack, and started my watch at that point. At most races everyone always starts out stronger than their race pace and then peters out, and this was no different. I figured I was hoping to run a 8:45 to 9:00 pace per mile, so I wasn't too surprised when the first mile went by in 8:23...even with passing a lot of people. The first two miles were on paved roads, and then transitioned to a metro park trail of crushed limestone. What did surprise me is that as the race progressed, I kept and average pace of about 8:20 per mile until about the 9-mile point. Because of the cool air, and the amount of moisture in the air, I noticed somewhere around the 5-6 mile point that my arms were coated with tiny little dew droplets that looked like little gems. I was wearing a black long sleeve shirt, so they really stood out. They stayed with me till the very end, although they were much fewer in number by the end. I still don't know if those were dewdrops or sweat beads that worked out through the shirt.

Although I chose not to listen to my mp3 player during the run, I think in the future I will. The chatter of other folks who are running with partners is somewhat distracting to me, and I think a little groove suits me just fine...like it does on training runs.

I had a pack of "sports beans" before the race, which are jelly beans with electrolytes in them, and was supposed to take an energy gel at about 45 minutes in and then another at 1 hour 30 min. I passed up the aid station at 38 minutes that had the gels, and figured we were turning around and would be passing back by there within 12-15 more minutes and I would get one then. WRONG. By the time I got back to that aid station they were out of gels, so I just got a cup of Gatorade and slowed down so I could drink the whole thing rather than slosh it all over myself like I do when I try to drink while running. The next aid station where I was able to get a gel was at about 1 hour and 15 minutes for me, and it was welcomed. The gels are an electrolyte replacement similar to what you get in a sports drink, but they are thick and come in a squeezable little pouch.

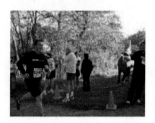

There were several stations along the way with folks cheering us on and some playing music, which really give a lift while running through those areas. Coming into the end was a relief as I was pretty drained from the exertion, but also felt very good when finished. I think my legs felt noticeably better than after a 13-mile training run I did, which I only ran in two hours ten minutes. My finishing time for today's half marathon was 1:52:44.95 (who's counting the .95? - can't we just call it 45 seconds?) Since my goal go into the race was pretty much just to finish it, and then if possible beat 2 hours.... I was very pleased.

My next adventure will be to run my very first marathon with Dean Karnazes, the famous endurance runner, on October 20. He is going around the country running 50 marathons in 50 states in 50 consecutive days (www.endurance50.com). I figure this may be only a once around time deal in my lifetime so I am going to make it my first marathon. The location and course is Cleveland, OH and should be the exact racecourse they use in the annual May marathon here. The pace, according to his website, should be around 4 hours 30 minutes, to 5 hours, which would suit me just fine, I just want to finish. But, if I don't, I still count it as a win, to have seen that I want to do it, and stepped up to the plate and give it a shot. I will train fully for a marathon next year, and hope to run either the normal Cleveland marathon, or the London, England marathon if I can get a slot to run that to benefit mental illness. There is an organization in England apparently called Mind, which offers slots to fundraising runners.

Chapter 3 – The marathon (and beyond?)

Runners could sign up to run with Dean (up to 50 runners per state of course) and for a fee run a supported small marathon and the proceeds go to charity. Could I do this? I was trying to decide and the question was burning me up around this time. His run in Cleveland near where I lived would be October 20, only 12 days after my first marathon. Could I possibly finish this? The answer came to me out of nowhere. It doesn't matter! I knew I wanted to try it, or I wouldn't have been thinking about it so much. If I showed up and only ran 18 or 20 miles, would I be a failure? NO. I would be a failure if I wanted to try it, and I was instead sitting on my couch that morning watching TV.

I signed up. Here is the blog post I made right after the marathon:

!!First Marathon!!

Friday, October 20th, 2006 I ran my first marathon as part of the Endurance 50, an event being run with Dean Karnazes an ultra famous ultra runner. I had really questioned the intelligence of trying to run my first marathon only 12 days after

running my first half marathon in the Towpath marathon here in Ohio. A while back when I was contemplating just this the thought occurred to me that the only failure I could suffer on this Friday would be to have this event going on and me sitting at home wishing I was there. I decided I was not concerned with whether or not I could finish the marathon, or how fast, so much as the fact that I had the courage to go out and try. I signed up.

There were a maximum of 50 runners allowed in each city to run the event with Dean, and my revelation allowed me to go ahead and sign up in time to be one of these 50. The morning of October 20 dawned to chilly temperatures of around 45 degrees and light rain. The check in for the event was set to begin at 0700 am at the corner of E 13th St. and St. Clair in downtown Cleveland, OH. This was also to be the start and finish line as it is in the normal Cleveland marathon. Because the marathons Dean is running are 50 in a row in 50 different states in 50 consecutive days, most of these events cannot fall on the same day as the "normal" marathon in that city. They are recreated marathons running the identical approved marathon course, but with only 50 runners. About 8 of Dean's marathons actually fall on the same day as the regular marathon, like his last event which falls on November 5, the same day as the NYC marathon, also being run by my friend Tyler Darby (www.aircrewphotos.com) and Lance Armstrong, the 7 time winner of the Tour de France (www.livestrong.org)

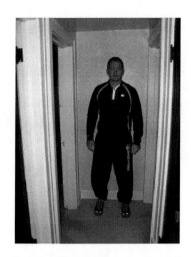

(Jazzed at 0530 am...let me run dammit!)

Naturally, I showed up around 0645 because I was so jazzed and didn't want to be late. In fact, I woke up about 5 times the night before, each time to be disappointed that I had so much time left to "sleep" away. I wanted to run!!!! Because of the inclement weather, we found ourselves congregating in the lobby of the Galleria mall, which happens to be right at that intersection. As I started to meet the runners, I found out that in the crowd was also a guy that I had gone to junior high and high school with, and hadn't seen in maybe 17 years. What a treat. I also ran into several people I had come in contact with via the internet in regards to the event. One guy, Joe Vasil, had contacted me through an ultra running web group on Yahoo and ended up being a big supporter of me through the run. It was said by many of the runners in the crowd this day, that this is perhaps the best possible environment that a runner could ever run their first marathon in, and now, after the fact, I know it too.

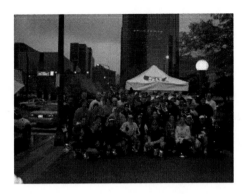

(I am in the upper left with green stripes on my sleeve.)

We took a few pictures before the event and started off close to on time at about 0800am running east down St. Clair. The tone of the day was to be more or less a "fun run" atmosphere, and that suited me just fine. We started off cold, getting a little wet, but excited and alert.

I had prepared my body as much as I could in the weeks before, tapering somewhat in the week before the run, by running less and trying to stretch when I could. I ate a big bowl of whole-wheat spaghetti the night before and drank plenty of fluids to make sure I would start the day well hydrated. I was plenty of hydrated.... I had to pull over and pee by the time we got to Cleveland Browns stadium, maybe 2 miles in. That should please any Steelers fans reading this blog, but it had no extra emotional appeal to me, because I am a Chargers fan. I would also stop to pee three other times during the run, but will have the good taste to describe those in less detail.

After the stadium pee I found myself a little behind the pack and as I caught back up, I hung out in the back with a gentleman who was running his own pace and not concerned with the pack leaving him behind. Turns out he is 62 years old, and runs about 5 miles per hour whenever he runs, but he can run that pace all day long. I enjoyed running alongside him, and wish I could remember his name and those of many other runners I met that day to include on this report. He was only running a half marathon this day, which was pretty easy on the Cleveland course because halfway into it you run back past downtown headed towards the east side and you can just drop off and go to the start/finish line. I learned so much from the runners I had the good fortune to suffer with this rainy cold Friday morning.

The first quarter of the run was honestly pretty easy and by the time we turned around at W. 117th street and started back towards downtown I was feeling pretty confident. I had run alongside my grade school friend Mack Bell for quite awhile and also the owner/proprietor of a local running store here in the area whose name is Vince (www.verticalrunner.com) The rain was not heavy by any stretch during the first half, but always enough to keep the street from drying and also our clothes. We had a support vehicle run by the endurance 50 which would pass up and down along the pack during the run to the point where you could get water, sports drink (Cytomax - good stuff) , energy bars, gels, bananas, and even Vaseline every couple miles or so while you were running. I was conscious of not getting dehydrated or running out of energy or glycogen in the muscles so I took in drink and fuel when I could get it, even though I hadn't gotten thirsty or hungry yet. I probably got a little over hydrated since I did have to pee so often, but I think in this run and this atmosphere that was better than under hydrated and suffering because of it.

I had my chance to talk to Dean somewhere during the second quarter of the run when I found myself near him and I really had two questions on my mind. #1 - Many people had asked him about his body and how he was holding up....I asked how much he missed his home. I know his family was with him day after day, but I know from traveling for a living, how much it sucks just to constantly be somewhere other than your own home. He said that the whole event was so exciting to him, that he really didn't miss his home too much, although he loves where he lives, but having his family with him made it easy to do the time on the road. #2 - I had read that one thing Dean thought about was running from San Francisco to Hawaii in a device called a "hydrobronc" or something similar, which in a nutshell is a human sized hamster wheel which floats on the water and gets propelled when you run inside it. My question was - Dean, have you thought much about running around the world? Dean didn't hesitate to say that he had, but that it was something he didn't feel he could do until his children were older. WOW. I find it easy to dream big, but to here him say he has though about it, and to know that if anyone can do it, he can.... well, it is a big notion to say the least. Obviously no one can just run around the world because of those pesky oceans.... but if you wanted to do an official distance that counted (similar to round the world flights) you could probably just run till you hit an ocean, and then move north or south enough until you can find land again at the same longitude on which you can run east/west.

A "BLISTERING" PACE

Well, with the wet weather and this being my longest run, I guess it was bound to happen. At about mile 12 (according to the other runners wearing GPS watches) I realized all of a sudden that I had a blister under my left foot. Only 14.2 miles to go. Well, I had already decided and declared that my motto for the day was to come from a quote I recently saw from Steve Prefontaine, a famous

University of Oregon runner: "Most people run a race to see who is fastest. I run a race to see who has the most guts."

I decided at this point in time that I wasn't going to talk about the blister and have it become anyone else's concern. My thought was more like, if I don't talk about it, it isn't as big a deal to anyone else, or to me. It worked. I worked with how I put my foot down and tried to minimize the impact on that spot of the foot when I could, but mostly, I just gritted my teeth and thought about other stuff. It was another learning experience in that I know now what it is like to keep going after feeling that. I learned after the run from others about a product called body glide that I will try on my next run of over ten miles to see if it helps all areas of chafing. I expect there is some good advice in the collective advice of the several runners who advised me about body glide and I am going to try it. For that matter, before I forget, I knew ahead of time about the possibility of bleeding nipples and I had shaved and band-aided mine to avoid this. Well, I got my first glimpse of the truth about this when I saw one guy at the finish area with a bloody spot starting at his right nipple and extending down his shirt. The band aids worked great for me. I find myself wondering what his feet looked like...Deans too for that matter, after running 33 marathons in the 33 days prior to ours.

I actually fell into a very nice pace as I focused on my foot over the next 8 or so miles and I found that whatever I did, I kept ending up right at the front of our pack just plodding along. It wasn't to be upfront and I mean this, but I just didn't want to change pace too much just to drop back, and then not feel as good as I was feeling with the stride I had going on. I was pretty much at the front during the whole return route along the shoreline, right up until we started coming into the city. This was somewhere around mile 23 or so, and I found that I needed to pull over a few times to stretch just a little to keep it going on. This seemed to work well for me, and as I got back into the running each time, I was able to keep with the pack and feel better for quite a while before having to do a little stretch again. My last stretch would come with about 1/4 mile to go, and had some of my good supporters (like Joe Vasil) concerned that I was pulling over to pull out.... not a chance. I just needed to stretch the hammies and kind of give my body a break from the constant position and alignment it was in while running mile after mile. I was finding that just bending over and kind of moving around a bit, would make me feel a lot better when I got back into the running stride and in the pack. Joe and several other runners were very helpful and vocal encouraging me to "just hang in there Mike, another little bit and you will have run your first marathon!" They don't know how much they helped! It was more than the spectators on the city streets or anyone else. They suffered through the last 25 miles with me, and they knew what a first marathon was like. Their encouragement definitely put a few extra strides into my legs to get me around the corner and keep me in the main pack.

I finished my first marathon (with the help of friends) in a "blistering" 4 hours and 19 minutes. When I finished this run, and more or less limped into the finish area back inside the mall, I really didn't feel like there was going to be more long runs like that in my future, but that was 26 miles of pain talking there.... I gotta say at this point, I am not done with this. I have something in my brain that probably won't let me go, so I am mentally preparing myself to start training for and then running the "Burning River 100." This is a 100 mile endurance run (let's not call it a race for me, I just want to see if I can do it in under a day) which will have it's inaugural running next summer August 4, 2006 in my area of Ohio (www.burningriver100.org) The start line is on the far east side of Cleveland and the finish line is about 10-15 blocks from my home in Cuyahoga Falls, OH. More to come on the training for this, and whether or not I am nuts enough to sign up, but right now, if I was betting, I would say...count on it.

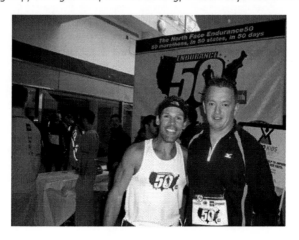

Ultramarathon Man Dean Karnazes and I at the Endurance 50.

So, now I have run a marathon. What next? I didn't really know. I knew I was charged up from meeting Dean, and I was going to keep running long distances. I had made the decision somewhere in here that I was going to attempt to run a 100 mile race the following summer. There was an inaugural race in my area called the Burning River 100, slated to be run August 4th and 5th. I decided, just like the marathon with Dean that I just had to sign up and see how it went.

My friend Tyler was set to run his first marathon at the NYC marathon on Nov. 5th and I told him I would like to be there to cheer him on and see him finish. I was off this weekend and arranged it so that I could travel to NYC and stay with very nice friends of the family on Staten Island, Larry and Patty.

Knowing I would want to run some the night before Tyler's marathon, I took running clothes and shoes. We got to Staten Island and Larry and Patty took my wife and I out for dinner at a nice place on the shore. We chatted about this and that, and intermixed in there was some talk about my marathon and my running and weight loss. I mentioned how I was going to run some on the island this night after dinner. Larry, with a mischievous glint in his eye, points out that I probably wished I was running the marathon with Tyler. It was kind of framed as part question and part statement. I didn't hesitate in saying yes, that if it were possible, it would be only too cool to be able to share this marathon with my friend. Larry asks if I mean it. Am I recovered enough? I state sure, and I was actually feeling fine. It had been two weeks since running the Endurance 50 marathon with Dean and the crowd and I felt great. "Did I really mean it?," Larry asked. Yes!

He whips out the cell phone and makes a call. A good friend and colleague of his, Joe Habib, runs the marathon every year and Larry knows that this particular year Joe cannot run it because he is proctoring a very important college entrance exam. He suspects that Joe is pre-registered as always and would have a bib number, and timing chip, etc. The phone call confirms as much, and that Joe cannot run the race, and would be happy to have me take his number and chip and run in his place. Oh, WOW!!!! So the whirlwind begins. I want some different socks for the marathon and we head to Target to get them. We drive into the city and get the bib and chip from Joe, leaving behind heartfelt thanks and promises to do well for him.

Many laughs ensue regarding the fact that I will be running the race as Joe Habib! Tyler is flabbergasted that I will be at his side instead of on the sideline and just so pumped! I will include the blog post here and you may see that Tyler had an even more exciting weekend than I....

YOU DID WHAT?

Well, this could be a long blog post. I went out to NYC with my wife to support my good friend Tyler Darby running in his first marathon. I planned on getting into position to take some good pictures, and just generally root him on in any way I could. We arrived to our friend's house on Staten Island on Saturday about noon to be in position.

I had packed my running gear so if the opportunity arose, I could go for a run on Staten Island, or even Central Park if we went into the city and I had a chance. After arriving on SI, we relaxed from the drive in for a little while before heading out to lunch. Prior to leaving for lunch I mentioned that I had brought my shoes, etc. and if my friend Tyler's team that he was running with, Team For Kids, had a runner go down for any reason I would be willing to step in and run the race.... just on a lark I told that to our friend we were staying with, Larry Ronaldson. He jumped on my comment and told me that they have a close friend who runs the NYC marathon every year, and this year he was unable to do so, because he had to do some unavoidable work that day, but that he had already gotten his race number and timing chip, etc. Did I want for us to call him and see if I could run in this guys place? Heck yeah, no hesitation.

We called, and left a message. This guy (I will omit his name, because I don't think the race looks kindly on runners having substitute runners) wasn't home and we had to wait until MUCH later in the day to see if this was even possible. Now keep in mind, that I had NO plans to run the race for real, so in the week prior to the race, I had run 20 miles on Thursday in the woods, and another 20+ miles earlier in the week. The race was on Sunday, for which one would normally "taper" off in the week or so prior to the race, so that the legs are well rested. Well, what can one do when you are training for a 100-mile race? You just can't think conventionally here folks. I had to view this as just another training run, or step along the way to the Burning River 100.

We went to lunch on Staten Island and then into the city to visit with Tyler, and as I found out, his new fiancé Kelley. Tyler had finagled his way into staying at a friends VERY nice apartment on the west side of Manhattan which was on the 42nd floor of the building facing the city and had a magnificent view....the city, central park, the statue of liberty, all was in sight.

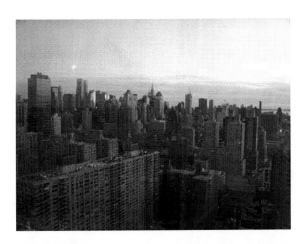

Tyler had proposed to Kelley with this view as the backdrop on Friday night with the city all blazing with lights. Man, what a good deal. I proposed to my wife in a Chinese restaurant. I know who did better on that one.

So we visited for several hours just enjoying everyone's company, and talking about the engagement and the marathon to come the next morning. When it was just about time to go and drop Tyler and Kelley off at a restaurant for dinner and drinks with his family, we finally got a hold of the runner who was not going to be running in the morning. Yes, he had his race bib, and timing chip, and yes, he would be happy to let me use them to run the race in his stead. The mood in the apartment, though already electric, jumped up just another notch. Tyler was so very excited that he was going to have a friend running with him. I was so very excited to be that someone. I had gone from running in probably the smallest marathon I ever will with Dean Karnazes on October 20 - my FIRST marathon - to running in the largest marathon in the world with 37,000+ runners. I had also run my first half marathon on October 8. So less than a month after my first half marathon, I ran two marathons.... crazy if you look at it ahead of time as a plan, but after the fact, I have no regrets.

After dropping off Tyler and Kelley we stopped to pick up the race packet on the way back over to Staten Island. It was kind of funny, because the drive in and back out of the city was very similar in routing to the route of the marathon. I got a lot of recon on the general lay of the course to be run the next morning. I learned why the 59th Street Bridge is called the groovy bridge, a point that would have me singing the 59th street bridge song as I crossed it the following morning. Listen to Simon and Garfunkels "59th Street Bridge Song" for more on that one, but I guess locals call it the "groovy bridge."

We got the packet and headed back to the house for a beautiful dinner of spicy shrimp with pasta, a salad, with toasted almonds, and Gatorade for me. I salted the pasta pretty strongly because I knew the next morning I would be losing a lot of salt via sweat. After dinner, we visited, and played chess...I set up the website to send my split times to my email and several friends. We went to Target so I could get some compression shorts and cheap gloves and a hat that I could discard as the race progressed and I warmed up.

I went to sleep around 10pm and planned on waking up at 630 am for a quick shower and bite to eat and then out the door to be dropped off around 8 am for the start at the Verrazanno Narrows bridge. I actually woke up at 0508 am and when I figured out where I was and remembered what I was getting up for this morning, sleep was all over...there was no way I could go back to sleep at this point. I got ready, had my shower...prepped everything I could for the race, like putting body glide on my feet, thighs, and nipples (found out later I should have also done my underarms...I had never chafed there before.) I also taped my nipples over to prevent chafing. For those reading this blog without long distance running experience, it is not uncommon for people running long distances to have their nipples rub against their shirts so much that by the end of a marathon, they are bleeding. I saw a pretty graphic example of this during my first marathon on a guy wearing a white shirt.... I wish I had a picture.

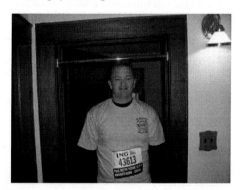

For breakfast/race prep I had a CLIF bar, a few pieces of pumpkin bread (homemade - and AWESOME, got the recipe for that one.) I drank a Gatorade. Heading over to the race start I carried some sports beans (essentially jelly beans with sodium and potassium added) and a caramel flavored gel. We could only get so close in the car, so about 1/2 miles from the start, I jumped out and walked/jogged the rest of the way into the start area for the race. Through talking with Tyler on a cell phone on the way in, I was able to find my way to him in the Team for Kids area at the start. Because we are not elite runners starting near the very front of the course, we could start and run together even though our designated starting areas were different. The NYC marathon has three different starting routes because of the extreme number of runners; they are color coded as blue, green, and orange. I was given green and Tyler was blue. Well, after we stretched and the 1010 a.m. start time was approaching, Tyler and I started walking towards the line and chatting along the way. We found the start but of course, since he was blue, and I was green, we wound up starting with the orange runners. Makes perfect sense right? Don't know how that happened, we thought we were headed to the blue start. No complaints though, this meant we would run over the top of the bridge vs. underneath on the second roadway down. MUCH better view.

Prior to the start we chatted with runners from all over. We saw folks from the Virgin Islands, Latvia, Belgium, Ireland, and Germany among others. At the starting line area, there were clothes coming off everywhere. People were discarding sweats, sweatshirts, hats, gloves...you name it. They were all tossed over near the side of the bridge. Word is that all this clothing is collected and given to charity once the runners depart. We were much closer to the front of the pack than we would have normally chosen so once we started out, we headed over to the left edge of the bridge and kept a pace set by Tyler's GPS watch. We were shooting for 10 minutes per mile.

Going over the bridge there were ships in the harbor, including two firefighting ships spraying water into the air like a mobile fountain. As we exited the bridge we could see one of the other colored routes coming off of the bridge and running a parallel route for a while. It was like a flood of runners just spilling into Brooklyn. As we hit the city streets, the sidewalks were filled with spectators shoulder to shoulder cheering on the runners. I very quickly was introduced to a beautiful way to hear verbal support in the longer, larger marathons. Tyler had written his name in large black letters on the front of his jersey (later I will tell you what he wrote on the back) and over the next 24 miles, I probably heard "Go Tyler!" and "Keep it up Tyler!" about 1000 times. That is no exaggeration. I won't forget that one. I tried to imagine my name was Tyler at some points in the race, just to mentally receive the encouragement.... ha.

The first 10 miles were pretty smooth. When it is chilly out, and I am well hydrated, I have to pee a lot, so only about 4 miles in, I had to pull off and pee. There were port o potties set up along the sidewalks, but everyone had like 8-9 runners waiting to use them, and I wasn't standing around to pee while everyone else kept running. I waited for a somewhat discreet street corner and dashed over to a fence to water South Brooklyn. Back onto the course, we were making good time on our ten minutes per mile pace. We even picked it up over the next mile to make up for the pee break.

27

Throughout the race we saw people running dressed as Elvis, a giant coffee cup, wearing all sorts of wigs (a bright blue one sticks out in my memory.) We saw people competing in wheelchairs. We saw one blind runner tethered to a sighted runner - how I would love to run a marathon for someone else as their guide! That would be very satisfying.

The aid stations were roughly every 2-3 miles with Gatorade and water. I have actually started to get decent a drinking from a cup while running without splashing it all over myself. Going into an aid station at about mile 6, they were very unprepared (the ONLY aid station I would say this about) but as they tried to quickly fill Gatorade cups and hand them out, it was ugly. Tyler grabbed the first cup offered him and then someone bumped him hard and the Gatorade went all down my right leg and shoe. Yuck. 20 more miles with a sticky leg and foot. Oh well.

I pitched my hat about mile 7 or so, and was going to pitch my gloves, but thought maybe I would want them later, so I put them in a pocket in my shorts.

As we got close to the end of our time in Brooklyn and Queens we started across one small bridge, which I mistakenly thought was the start of the 59th Street Bridge, so I started singing the Simon and Garfunkel song. Immediately, there were 10-15 other runners joining in....we only sang maybe the first four lines, but it was a very fun moment for me. I didn't expect the accompaniment.

Feeling pretty decent we hit the real 59th street bridge around mile 15 with the expectation that Tyler's Mom, new fiancé, and brother Grant would be waiting for us on the other side before we headed north through Manhattan. It was kind of weird starting across the bridge because for a while you are running in the dark. For maybe 1/8 mile or so. I sang the song again at this point with little to no help from others...We started down the left side of the roadway on the bridge, but somewhere over halfway we transitioned to the right so we would be one the side we expected Tyler's family, and possibly my wife. As we ran downhill on the right side of the bridge, I looked down and saw that someone had discarded a Fuel Belt. This is a elastic type belt made to hold small water bottles and stuff for longer runs. I had wanted one for my longer runs, but didn't buy one yet, because they aren't cheap and I didn't NEED it yet. I made a comment to Tyler that I should have picked it up about 100 yards later, and he said "Go back and get it!" So I did. I turned around and ran against the flow for about 100 yards and snagged it and then blasted back down the edge to meet Tyler. As we exited the bridge, the route takes us around a 270-degree turn at the end of which we found Tyler's crowd. My wife hadn't made it yet through the city. We stopped for about two minutes and Tyler told his mom, that someone had written something on the back of his shirt as we ran. When he turned around to show her, his shirt simply said, "Kelley said Yes." His mom new right away and was very pleased. She was also surprised to see me, because we hadn't told her I would be running with Tyler. I handed off the fuel belt to Kelley who gave it to my wife and we headed off north along 1st avenue. Somewhere in the next 5 miles headed north is where I started to feel the effects of running all those miles in the 6 days before this marathon. I just put it out of my mind and hung on next to and behind Tyler.

At the very northern end of this leg, we turned around in the Bronx and then headed south down through Harlem and then the eastern side of Central Park. Heading south, I was really feeling tired of running and wanted to suggest doing like a one-minute walk/ 5 minute run rotation to Tyler. Somehow I kept my mouth shut and just kept placing one foot in front of the other. I would say at this point, I felt the same as the last few miles of the Dean marathon, but I just kept going on. We ran into Coach Adam from Team for Kids and he gave us a little mental trick to help us through some of the shallow up hills to come. I also had another mental image given to me from our host Larry Ronaldson that helped to distract me from what I was feeling and just let me keep running. He practices Tai Chi and gave me an energy demonstration the night before that I turned into a visual image for running.

Tyler was bullet proof and I really felt like he could have run away from me at any point if he wanted to. As we entered Central Park I was somewhat energized by the sight of familiar territory as I have run through there before. I got some energy back headed down the east side. As we rounded the southern end and headed west, we were caught up for quite awhile looking for Tyler's family as they were supposed to be along the side waiting for us. We never did see them, but we pressed on across the southern end and then at Columbus Circle turned north for the last leg into the finish line. As we passed the grandstand along the way in, I was lucky enough to see my wife and Patty Ronaldson in the stands rooting me on. Afterwards my wife would tell me that we looked like we had plenty of energy at this point and were running well. Boy did we fool her! I was just depleted and running mostly on will at this point.

In the last few hundred yards, I had already made the decision that I would love to finish side by side with Tyler, but if he kicked and sprinted in, I was just watching him. This was his weekend, and even if I had it in me (questionable) I wasn't racing him to the line. He finished three seconds and about 30 feet in front of me! Tyler: 4:20:53 Me: 4:20:56. Pace per mile: 9:57.

As I slowed back to a subsonic speed crossing the finish line I must say that although the running itself wasn't much easier than my first marathon 16 days prior, the recovery immediately after the race was much more agreeable. After the first marathon I felt very wobbly on my legs and like my knees were puffy with fluid, but this day I was mostly just sore, but much more comfortable walking around and standing. We first hit the handout of the medals as we progressed through the finish area. Next came the Mylar blankets, which were taped around us to keep the body heat in. Shortly after that came the much needed water and Gatorade. As we progressed along we looked for the Team for Kids area, and there was someone checking you through the gate by looking for a TFK shirt. I didn't have one and was going to be forced to go off alone until I made the guy realize Tyler was my ride and contact point to find a way home. Then he relented and let me in.

We got cell phones and made contact with Kelley who came to meet us, and then found out where my wife was, and the rest of the family and met them outside of the park at 72nd street and Amsterdam. We exchanged stories and congratulations...took some pictures and then headed out our separate ways. I wanted to try to make it to the Endurance 50 wrap-up event at the North Face Store on Broadway, which ended at 4pm. I got there at about 3:55pm and was unable to see Dean but I nabbed some nice goodies from the sponsors.

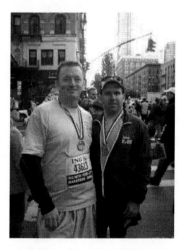

We headed a few blocks away and got some New York pizza. I had two slices of pepperoni and drank some vanilla protein milks I had scored from the Endurance 50 thing. The protein right after workouts supposedly helps the muscles start to recover.

Just as a wrap-up, the very next night back in Ohio, a friend called that I had told I would run with when I didn't know I was doing the marathon. We went out and ran 10.2 miles on the Buckeye Trail at night, which was my first night trail running experience. I learned a lot this night about running trails in the dark and found out I needed a stronger headlamp for it. The greatest thing about these runs is seeing the eyes shining out from the woods around you and trying to figure out what kind of animal it is. We saw 13 deer this night....one as close as 30 feet or so.

Chapter 4 – So can I be an "ultra marathon" man?

My initial plan to make myself ready for the challenge of 100 miles, was to add 10 miles to my longest run each month between this timeframe and the race the next summer. Experienced runners who had run these "ultramarathons" (races longer than marathons) would soon talk me out of this plan.

Later this November, I conceived of the perfect opportunity to get a very long run in, as Thanksgiving was here and we always go to my parent's house. They live about 27-28 miles away depending on the route I use to get there. One of the key planning aspects of this run, which is not in the following blog post is that I told my Dad how I was getting there, but NOT my Mom. He knew enough to keep it from her until I arrived. You would have loved the look on her face when she realized how I got to her house for Thanksgiving dinner. Here we go again:

How do you get to the Turkey?

So, in keeping with my plan to add 10 miles each month to my long run (which I may modify based on the advice of a fellow ultrarunner with a lot of experience) I decided today was the day to complete my 30 miles distance for November. I had tried last Sunday night to get the distance in by running the course of the Buckeye Trail 50k with Brian Musick, but when we got into the trails it was raining and snowing, and the ground was so slippery we had to walk in many places we would normally be running...just for safety. We were making terrible time, and both were kind of miserable so we exited the woods at about 9 miles and ran back via roads and towpath to the car for a total distance of 14.2 miles.

I ran from my house in Cuyahoga Falls to my parent's house in North Lawrence, OH. The distance I was planning was 32-33 miles based on mapping it out on the internet. I ended up running 27.9 miles because I was feeling really tight in one of my legs and cut the last portion shorter and took a more direct route to get there.

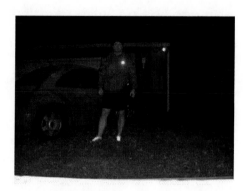

I arose at 5:20 am to get ready and took longer than expected, but still got out the door at 6:38 am. The temperature was 25 degrees F at the time I left the house. Projecting I would get in sometime around noon the temps were supposed to be 47 degrees by then. I wore my Mizuno shoes, regular socks, compression shorts under Brooks running shorts, a high tech type t-shirt (short sleeve), and a light jacket I just got which has a pocket for the mp3 player. Definitely chilly to even cold to start off, but I was hoping to be comfortable later in the run without having to discard clothing. There was frost all over the ground and cars as I went outside, and the sun was just starting to tint the horizon green and blue.

Leaving my neighborhood, I ran under a large Christmas tree as I got onto the main road. Getting into downtown Akron, I was trying to watch signs for the towpath connection (the trail I was trying to follow) but about halfway through town they just disappear. I saw the path at the back of a park and headed back in to reconnect with my trail, but then it was blocked off because they haven't finished the whole length...so I retraced my steps back out to the main road. I little later I connected the trail again, only to have to detour back out to the main road when the trail ended before reaching the edge of town.

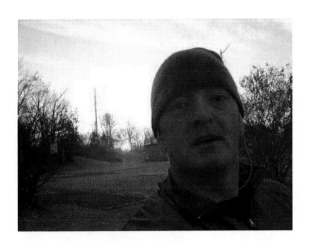

The first 15-18 miles or so were pretty uneventful....felt good....just putting em down one after the other, but around 18 miles or so, I started to feel some discomfort behind my left knee....I am assuming the hamstring. I slowed up to ease it and it helped some, but then even that didn't help so I started walking...and stopping and stretching it out and massaging it. I would be able to run for about 100 yards at a time after each stretch, but it would come right back, and I was starting to think that I was going to have to walk all the way to my parents (which I was fine doing, even though I would be much later than planned.) side note: I did NOT tell my mom I was running down because she would spend the entire morning worried. She doesn't fully get the idea that she should be worrying about me when I stop doing these crazy stunts.....that is when I am in trouble. The fact that I am out there doing something I dreamed up, just means I am doing good.

Anyways after several miles of the walk run thing, I remembered I had brought a little energy drink thingy along. It is packed full of Vitamin B12 and caffeine....so I thought that it couldn't hurt. I wanted to see if I would get an energy boost anyhow. I sucked it on down, and after about two more iterations of the walk run thing, I noticed the pain disappearing so I just kept running.

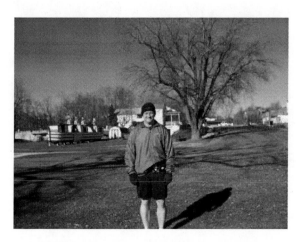

The calorie counter I use states that I would have burned around 4900 calories on this run for my weight. Even though I ate a nice Thanksgiving meal, I didn't come anywhere near replacing these calories today. I still ate healthy with turkey, stuffing, corn, coleslaw, and diet soda. Oh yeah, also some pumpkin bread that I made with Splenda instead of sugar.

The next step in my journey to run 100 miles was that I would show up and run an event called an FA 50. This particular FA 50 was called Art Moore's FA because he organizes it and has been a successful runner in our area for some time. What is an FA? Well, FA is the acronym for Fat Ass and is named such because they are typically run during the holidays to keep one from getting such an ass.

Most people were going to run 50 kilometers (31 miles) this day, but Kurt Osadchuk and I felt compelled to go 50 miles in the interest of being ready for the 100 miler. The story as I saw it went:

I kept going and going and going....

Felt like I was a rabbit pounding away on a drum at times. I did my first 50 miler Saturday. Kurt and I arrived at the Scenic Park Trailhead of the Rocky River Reservation at around 0615am to start our 50-mile attempt and we met up with Kim Love of the Mohican Trail discussion group by chance. She was there to do 41 miles because it was her 41st birthday. After I gave her the birthday present I brought her, a pair of trail socks, we headed out at 0626am to start the journey.

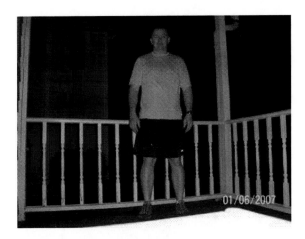

This picture is of me before leaving the house to drive up to Cleveland.

Because of all the recent rains here in Ohio, the river running through the parks (the Cuyahoga River) was swollen to the point of overflowing its banks, and blocking most, if not all of the sections of the biking and running trail we had wanted to use for the run. We quickly found out that we would have to run on the street to complete our day, and even then we would only be able to go about 3 miles before the water made the street impassable. On the first circuit out, we elected to turn around at 2 miles because we needed to get back to the parking lot at 0700am to meet up with our friends Cindy and Roger who were going to run with us for a while. Kim had a friend named Tom coming out to run with her as well. It turned out that 2 miles out would be the turn around all day long. This put us back at the car every 4 miles or basically once an hour, where we could eat, drink, or resupply anything. There is Kim, the birthday girl, getting ready to start her 41 miles. Look at that grin, even though she knows what she is going to feel like in 10 hours or so...wow.

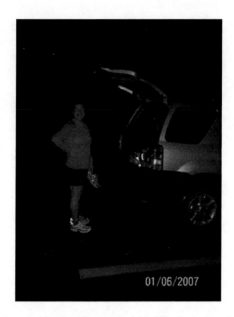

01/06/2007

We kind of got into a habit of taking around 10-12 minute breaks each time back to the car, which was a bit long. They were fine at first, but as I got more tired throughout the day, it got harder to start it back up after cooling down for that long. As I would find out on the last three circuits, when I was ultra tired and just wanting to get done, I did a lot better with basically no break. I stopped just long enough to pee at the toilet and grab water or Gatorade and head right back out. After the entire run was over, I got some good advice from Roy Heger about not getting too comfortable during breaks while running ultras, he says "beware the chair!" Although we didn't have chairs, I got his meaning, and will be trying to limit my breaks in future ultras.... not to finish faster, but to feel better hopefully during the whole run.

When Cindy and Roger graciously arrived at 7am to share a few miles with us, it was nice to see friends and have some discussion over the 12 miles that they would run with us. I won't forget how rewarding it was to have different people to talk with. Next summer when I attempt the 100 mile race (or races.... we will see) we will be allowed to have a "pacer" or someone running with us, after 60 miles in, and I hope that Roger, Cindy, Jim, or Debi will come out and run some with me. At that point in that run, I will probably be nearly delirious with exertion so I hope they will remember that when I am talking crazy....

After we had run nearly 12 miles with Cindy and Roger, Cindy's IT band started to give her a little warning to shut it down (she has recovered from an IT band injury.) Well, they ran in the last loop of their three loops and after our short little break and a photo, we took off running again and they drove home. Thanks Roger and Cindy!

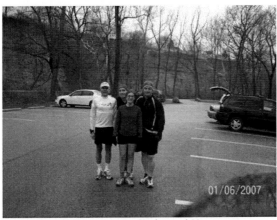

Kurt, **Roger**, Cindy, and **Me**

By the time we got to halfway (25 miles) at 5:30 both Kurt and I were feeling pretty good, and pretty confident. We had another break right at the 25-mile mark, so we didn't finish the marathon until 5:44, even though it was only 1.2 miles later. At this point in the run, I was feeling pretty confident that this thing was possible for me. I even said something to that effect. At the 50k or 31-mile mark we were at 6:36:54 and still feeling pretty positive. This was the first time I had run 50k in one stretch. I will be running a 50k on January 27th called the Winter Buckeye Trail 50k.

Now I have read that during ultra runs there are always low points and high points and you just have to weather the low and eventually things will look up, and you will go back into cruising mode. My low hit me right around the 34-35 mile mark when we were running along and I just kind of started feeling like I couldn't do this anymore. I told Kurt I needed to walk a short stretch and we walked about 2 minutes before we started back up and ran that loop all the way back to the car. After our break at the car, I was feeling like warmed over cat shit. I was giving serious consideration to just sitting down in the car and waiting for Kurt to finish, or even finding a way to go to the dinner that was going on over at **Colleen Theusch's** place. I mean, I could rationalize it by the fact that I did go 4 miles or so past the 50k, which I hadn't even ever done before.

Well it occurred to me that I would be giving up without even walking very much, and I had said that I would finish the damn 50 miles even if I had to walk

37

it out. We headed out from the car running, and after about a half mile, I found I needed to start walking again. Kurt went on running because he was feeling pretty good. He had done 50 miles before so I think he was more prepared. As I started walking, I found out something new about ultra running and me. After walking a little while, things would get sore, like my feet and legs, just from the walking.... and it would feel BETTER to run for a while. So for the next 10 miles or so, I would walk for about 5 minutes and then run for about 10 minutes. This actually kept me on nearly the same pace I had been doing when I was just running. I was still on pace to break 12 hours for the 50 miles, which was a goal I was hoping for, and Kurt was barely gaining any extra ground on me, even though I was mixing in the walking. Another thing I mixed in, which I mentioned before, was now that I was alone; I stopped taking the breaks back at the car. Just a quick squirt at the toilet, and grab something to drink at the car, and back out for the run/walk.

When I was coming back in around 41-42 miles or so, I ended up meeting back up with Kim and Tom for a mile and a half or so, and I ran this entire stretch back into the car with them, which finished her 41 miles (Kudos to you Kim! Great run!) She is also experienced at this and has done 62 miles before in one stretch. Well, after gutting it out with them, I realized I could run more than I thought and I decided to run a higher percentage of the rest of my run. My walking breaks went down to like 2-3 minutes, and I was making really good time. I could clearly see I could break 12 hours, and if I wanted to really open it up, I thought there was an outside chance that I could come in just under 11 hours. Well, that wasn't to be, because as I considered how I felt, I decided that the smarter thing to do was keep up what was working and be happy with the sub 12 which was my original goal. Strangely enough, it didn't seem to be that I didn't have enough energy; it was more a factor of the soreness in my ankles and thighs. I kind of felt like if I pushed my pace and tried to break 11 hours; my legs and joints would not handle it. Side note: I really need to start stretching better and more.

On the subject of creaky joints and whatnot, once I was running alone, I had a fun little realization. I kept getting mild paranoia when I would hear some of the gravel I would kick up or sticks I would step on and break, that this was my ankle or knee cracking or making noises. I realized after a while that my body wasn't making noises, but for a little bit, I was mildly worried that I was pushing myself too hard, until I realized where the noise was really coming from. When I was running with Kurt we were talking so much, and he had his music on, that I really didn't hear that gravel and sticks...

OK, homestretch. When I got to about 46 miles, I just really wanted to be done, so I decided to abandon the walk and try to finish out running. This turned out to be just fine, so I finished my first 50 miles in 11:22:43. Kurt had finished ahead of me in 10:59:23 and since he was trying to get more mileage anyhow, he kept going while I was finishing and he ran a total of 52 miles. Also, the nut job (I say this in fun) went home to the local gym and ran another 1.25 miles before calling it a night. He was going to try to get 65 total miles in all. He may have even woken up this morning to crank out another 10-11 miles before 626am to fulfill that goal...who knows? Since he broke his personal best in the 50 miles by 5 hours, I hope he just slept in.

After I thought about it awhile, I figured I would add some information at the end of this post. First is a hearty thanks for the volunteers who set up and provided the excellent hot dinner at **Colleen Theusch's** house after our run Saturday. They are also the volunteers who give of their time every summer at the Mohican 100 trail race in Loudonville, OH. I want to run that race more just because they will all be there taking care of us!

Second was that I thought it would be interesting to detail my nutrition for the day of my 50 mile run. When I woke up that morning, I had a bowl of instant (sugarless) oatmeal...two packets. I also drank a Myoplex vanilla protein drink. On the drive up to Cleveland I had an Oats and Honey Granola bar (Nature Valley) and a diet mountain dew.

I went through two packs of Clif Shot blocks, one apricot Clif bar, three peanut butter and jelly sandwiches, three Gatorades (20oz.), two propel fitness waters, three more Myoplex vanilla protein drinks (the last one after I was done to help recovery start...), three Endurolite salt capsules, two pretzel sticks, and a handful of BBQ potato chips during the run. Every time we ate, the red squirrels of the Rocky River Reservation kept themselves VERY close at hand in case we dropped anything or fed them. Many people were tossing them bits of food, which is why I am sure they are so brave.

We got rained on lightly twice but never really bad. There were moments of sunshine, moments of rain, but mostly it was overcast all day.

Chapter 5 – Is it OK to fail sometimes?

Now, remember how when I started talking myself into these crazy long runs, I had told myself that if I had to stop short sometimes, I shouldn't feel like a failure? I was about to come smack up against that and see if I could practice what I was preaching. Though there are many days of running in between the races and longer events, I choose here to hit the highlights. My blog has details of many of the training runs leading up to these long runs.

I signed up for the Winter Buckeye Trail 50k, which is a 50-kilometer trail race in January run primarily in memory of a local running legend named Regis Shivers. It is run on a different course than the Summer BT50k, but in the same area and on some of the same trails.

WBT50k becomes WBT26m

(yes, I am dorky enough to use the blue blazes color for my post!)

All week long I was preparing myself mentally and in terms of gear for a brutally cold 50k run for Saturday. As the day got closer, it became more obvious that it wasn't going to be all that cold. The start of the race was at or near 40 degrees F and the temp only gradually dropped off during the day. I started out with a balaclava from The North Face on and a set of Columbia skiing gloves. Just a mile or two in it was obvious that this was excessive and at the first pass back by the Boston Store (5 miles in) I stopped and dumped them off in my backpack. The rest of the day I would go without hat or gloves, which was comfortable as long as I was moving at a good pace.

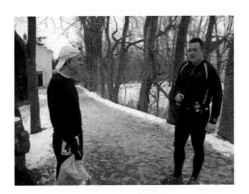

This is Kurt and I at the half marathon point.

Going into the race, I was prepared for the worst of trail conditions with extremely screwed shoes. I had added six more screws to the bottom of each of my shoes, and even added 9 double sets of lock washers under some screws to help grip snow and ice better. I also lost 12 screws during the race, most notably, almost all the screws off of the edge of the right heel. I even saw one of my lock washers on the ground the second time I was heading through the pine tree section on Pine Lane (PL) trail. Here are the pictures:

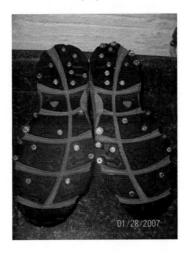

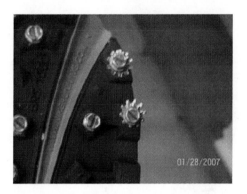

Now I thought this was a pretty damn clever innovation on a fairly simple technique for adding traction for inclement weather running. Indeed the washers did seem to add quite a bit of bite to my running. On several downhill sections I was just blazing past folks who were picking their way slowly down icy and slushy patches. It also added some considerable bite to my ankles. Notice how the washer extends out past the rubber in that second photo? This is called **"M**ad **S**cientist with **N**o Fore**S**ight **S**yndrome," more commonly referred to as MSNFSS (sounds like Muss N Fuss.) That damn little washer bit into my ankle several times during the day as my legs got tired and my feet would accidentally clip my inner ankle. If you decide to try the lock washers some day, pay attention to the clearance on the insides of the shoes so you don't do what I did! I don't think that this affected my running, but it sure was irritating and now I have a little wound to heal down there...

Back to the running, I was doing quite well during my first 13 miles; in fact I was a good bit ahead of where I thought I would be time wise. I don't think I was pushing my pace really though. I was still walking the up hills and jogging what felt comfortable to me on the flats and down hills. Occasionally on the down hills I would kind of let go and just let gravity pull me down. This may take out more energy than I realize, I don't know. I finished the first thirteen miles in 2:44, but had thought it would take me a solid 3 hours. Kurt O had really blazed out fast and did his first 13 in 2:13 I think, but then his knee starting hurting real bad and he had to call it quits. I felt bad for him, but when I saw him when I came in for 13 miles, I was already uncertain as to whether I could complete all 31 or not.

I pushed on out of Boston Store and headed up to Brandywine Falls (BF.) I took it easy as I was already hurting some and I walked for a little while drinking some hot chocolate I had put into a water bottle at BS. When I got to BF, I saw Roy Heger again and thanked him for the excellent trail markings and was reminded of how he taught me to "Beware of the Chair" when he told me their aid station motto was "Get the hell outta here!" I like it! I am starting to learn what works for me on long runs, and stopping for much time does not. I grabbed a PBJ quarter, some almonds and cashews and followed the motto.

Coming back again to BS, I was feeling pretty crappy, but not rock bottom so I knew I was going to Pine Lane and back at least for the marathon distance. I was rewarded as I neared BS by the sight of my two daughters building a snowman along the towpath, and I stopped and got some kisses. My wife brought some tomato soup (I had kinda requested/hinted/suggested this...) I then felt bad that I could only drink about a half inch of it out of a bowl after requesting it. I just had a funny stomach at that point.... not nauseous, but my appetite was low. I headed out for Pine Lane (PL) on more time.

Last week when we were previewing the BF trail, I took some enjoyment from listening to the trees moan and creak as they swayed in the winter wind. Shortly after heading back out for PL I decided I had listened to enough music for today and stowed my mp3 player. Not long afterwards, I started to delight in hearing nature sounds once again. The trees were groaning once again and I was enjoying it...oh wait...is that the trees? No, there wasn't enough wind. What I was hearing turned out to be my race number fluttering around behind me as it was strapped to my fuel belt. At least I got a good laugh at myself. I must have ran for about a mile thinking I was listening to the trees before I realized I was just hearing my own race bib.

The going was not comfortable. I have had some tenderness or soreness in my lower abs this week. I think it arose because I did a strenuous abs workout on Tuesday and then followed that by playing basketball. I could tell playing basketball that I shouldn't have been, but like many a young dumb gun, I played on because I love it. That is one of my weaknesses, that I LOVE playing basketball. Full court or half, I love to play in the game. I also had small stretches where my left heel kind of acted up like it did last week when I did the adventure night run. It would go away though, and I have been stretching it more since I have finished.

Somewhere around mile 19-20 after heading back for PL, my confidence in my screw shoes bit me. I was going downhill alongside some stairs and instead of being icy or snowy it was muddy, and WHAMMO I was on my butt. I laughed it off and went on, but more carefully. Heading back out on PL trail, I was probably only running 25% of the time. I would just run as much as I could and then back off to a walking pace. At the PL trailhead/aid station Kim caught back up to me and although we headed back out together for a half-mile or so, I just couldn't keep running with her and had to watch her go on. I did however shout several times as she motored on for her to "Go Get em!" I hope that helped. She is a strong runner and only getting better from what I hear. She is really a pleasure to run with, and although she has coined the term "ultra whining" on her blog, it must be an internal dialog, because I never hear it from her.

Somewhere in hear I also have to fit in a tribute to Bob Combs, Jim Harris, and Bill "Shubi" which is a nickname though I don't know his last name. They started out at 10pm the night before and ran the old winter 50k course before starting the current one with us. WOW, holy shit WOW! Jim was very strong and finished the entire 100k! Not to out Bob and Bill, but I saw them finishing their 44th mile when I was headed out for PL and they said they were done and going home. They have been very gracious with their advice and including me on some runs, and to see veterans like these calling it a day earlier than they had planned, only helped me to make the right decision.

I just did what I could coming back out of PL and though I wavered back and forth on the decision, I eventually decided it was in my best interest to just complete the marathon this day. I have learned, and am proud of the fact that my *ego* didn't injure my *body*. There is always a line to watch when running these distances, and I am proud that I stayed conservative this day. Coming down out of PL, I manufactured one last goal to accomplish. There was one runner a few hundred yards back on the trail and I decided if I wasn't going to do the last 5 miles, I was at least going to dig in a little bit and hold him off. He had been catching up to me for some ways. I did everything I could and ran the last 1/4 to 1/2 mile into BS and kept him at bay. My marathon time for the day was 6:28. So to make the math painfully obvious that was a 2:44 first 13 miles and a 3:44 second 13 miles.

I do have one big regret. I wish I could have passed through BF aid station one more time to express my thanks to the volunteers there for what they do. I really hope that I can volunteer at some races in the future and help be part of the machine that makes this all work!

No doubt this little "failure" if you can call it that, would weigh on my mind somewhat for awhile. Was it the slippery conditions? Was it my conditioning? Did I have a problem with my hips that would always slow me down? In the end, after a few weeks of reduced activity I felt back to normal from some of the issues that caused me pain this day. I kept running, but shorter distances and so on. I mixed in a lot of swimming in these weeks and weight lifting. I never saw the doctor (later I would wish I had...) but things got better.

I would have many assorted fun events (I came to call them "adventure runs") over the next months. I started a little game where I was seeing how many airports I could run around while I was on the road. I ran around some pretty big ones like Intercontinental Houston and Dallas Fort Worth. I learned some things about fueling myself during long runs on these adventures. I learned what the "bonk" truly feels like; when you have basically depleted your bodies glycogen stores and are running on "empty." The body cannot metabolize energy fast enough from fat to make running in this state comfortable and one generally slows down and slogs along. I have been there.

I did a run one afternoon in Santa Barbara, CA trying to get some hilly trails in and scared the crap out of myself when I came across some LARGE footprints on the trail at a point where it was pretty much a wash whether to turn around or go forward and finish in terms of distance.

My mentality going forward now was going to focus on two goals. I was going to focus on trying to run a good marathon at Cleveland in May, and then really focus on training up to the Burning River 100.

The immediate goal for the Cleveland marathon was to break 4 hours, and although I kept that in my mind, I never focused exactly on a training program specifically for the marathon. I did my runs in a "whatever I feel like" kind of style. Even though my good friend Tony advised me to get into his preferred marathon training book, I kind of just figured if I kept putting in a good amount of mileage, that I could count on doing what I wanted.

I had many fun adventures in March...

Chapter 6 – "Adventure" Running

This and That

First off, today I got a *really* cool email. I had asked Kim (I call her Mohican Kim) about how she got the cool picture at the top of her blog, and she replied with instructions on how to do what you see above. Then she went on to tell me she is working the aid station sponsored by the NEO (NorthEast Ohio) trail group, of which I am a member, at mile 65 on the Burning River course AND she plans on dropping her duties there when I show up, and running with me as a pacer! I am so honored. As Kim mentions on her <u>blog</u>, we have very similar attitudes and got along great when we ran together for some of the Winter Buckeye Trail 50k. I think her pink dirty girl gaiters hypnotized me for some part of the run and I just kept a'following them ankles.

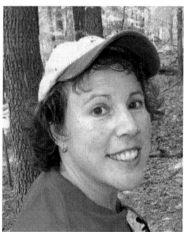

Thanks Kim!

I am also planning on providing pacing/company for her during the Mohican 100 in June. I hope I serve her well, it will be my first time as a pacer, and I think it will be a good decision for me to just run part of that race by pacing instead of trying to do two 100's my first year. If I finish BR100, my reward will be to run both races in 2008, and if I finish both of them, then I will reward myself in 2009 with a "big" race either out west, or even Mountain Masochist.

OK, on to a few other items. I bought a new camera. 7.2 megapixel Casio Exilim which is VERY compact and will be even easier for me to carry on runs and while traveling. The old one was a 5 m.p. Kodak, which still works and will be a backup in case I have problems. I just found a deal I couldn't resist on a floor model of the Casio, so I got it.

I made this collage of my face about a month ago, and can't believe I didn't think of putting it on here til today, but here it is on the next page. I also plan on making a smaller one to use as a header at the top of the page sometimes.

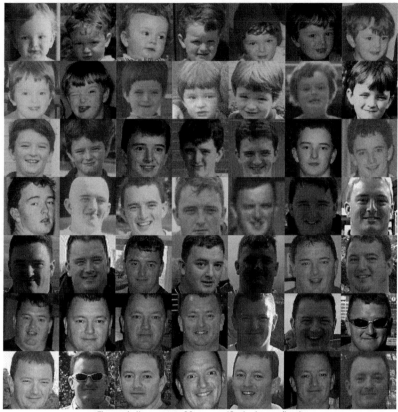

Through the years...33 years, 49 photos....yikes!

Oh yeah, what the hell did I do today exercise-wise? Swam 1/2 mile at 530am, lifted, shot a few baskets. Home all day being domestic. Back to the gym at 900pm, lifted, played hoops for an hour, ran a mile (6:59 - first timed mile since I started getting back in shape....) lifted a little more, and then home to type this. Got to go sleepie bye now. Good night!

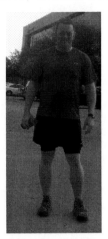

DFW (Dallas Fort Worth) Perimeter Run

I have been largely silent for several days because my hotel in Los Colinas changed all the room modems, and can't seem to get the internet back up and running.

Saturday, after class, I departed the Simuflite center to run around the perimeter of the DFW airport, a run which I had mapped out and figured to be 18.9 miles. I brought one water bottle filled with Gatorade and some cash in case I needed food or more liquids along the way. The time of departure from the Simuflite parking lot was 5pm or so.

Heading south out of the drive, it wasn't long before I had to stop and tie my shoe....when I was bent down tying it, a moth landed right near me so I shot him. Here is the result.

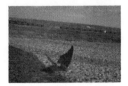

When I go out on longer runs, it seems as if the hardest miles are always the first few, and maybe the last few...somewhere in the middle everything seems easy and I just float along. I motored on around the southern edge of the airport on Airfield Drive, listening to some tunes to help drown out all the airplane noise, and the noise of all the cars driving by. When I have been running around the airports it does make me wonder whether it would be safer taking my chances on the trails with the possibility of a bear encounter, or dodging some of the wacko drivers that I see out there. Now that I have made a friend who is an insurance underwriter (you know who you are) maybe that person can do an assessment for me and let me know what would be smarter! As I headed up the east side, on East Airfield Drive, I took this photo and.....

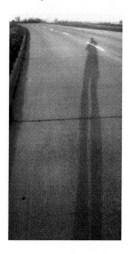

right about here is where I goofed up missed a turn. I went maybe a mile up East Airfield drive before I realized I was between the runways, and had to backtrack that mile if I wanted to be able to say I did the entire perimeter run. I stopped for maybe a minute and just stood there for a minute, just pondering whether I should turn back or just head on...but I turned back.

My plan had been from the beginning to carry one water bottle filled with Gatorade, and drink from it...about 9 miles in, which was halfway until I added the little side trip, there is a convenience store, where I was going to get another Gatorade and eat some food to keep me going. For some reason when I got to that store, I figured I wasn't too hungry yet, and kept going...there was another store I knew of about

3-4 miles down the road, so that would be an option.

I headed across the North end of the airport, with another minor side trip by accident, but not as much of a mileage add-on as the first one, and when I got to the area on the other side of the field, I still wasn't too hungry, and I had found a water fountain to fill up my water bottle, so I thought I would save my money and just run back to my car, and then eat back at the hotel. STUPID. From this point on, I had maybe 4-5 miles to the car, and it just got progressively harder....I wasn't really sore, but just kind of hit a spot where I didn't want to run...hard to explain. I wasn't out of breath, I wasn't hurting...I think I was just low on glycogen stores and my body was trying to tell me to cut it out. I ended up walking off and on for the rest of the journey. It actually felt better when I would run, but after a little while I would end up walking some more. I think the real solution here is when I go on runs longer the 8-10 miles, I need to be eating 500-750 calories per hour to keep my energy up so I can keep up the pace for the entire run. I made the circuit of the airport in around 3 hours and 30 minutes but am confident that without going the wrong way, and fueling myself properly I can go around this airport in maybe 2 hours and 45 minutes, so maybe I will have do another loop sometime soon.

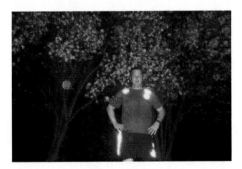

I have another one to come soon, because I ran around the perimeter of White Rock Lake last night with a fellow pilot...it was beautiful...9 miles...I will write it up soon.

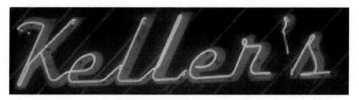

White Rock Lake (North of Dallas, TX)

Monday I was planning to run the trail or path around White Rock Lake in Dallas, TX when I got a pleasant surprise. Erik Barr, who flies for the same company as me, and was in class down here as well, is a runner and wanted to go along. After getting done with out training for the day, we both met back at the hotel and headed out for the lake, which was approximately 30 minutes drive away.

I was particularly excited because I got to wear my new "ugly" Brooks Cascadias. I was really anxious to see if they felt as good running as they did just trying them on. The good news is that they fit and felt great during the run, but I didn't get as much dirt time on them as I thought I would. The path around the lake is not a trail, but instead a paved bike/running trail. I ran as much as I could on the side of the path in the grass and dirt, but some places it wasn't practical, or there was too much of a side slope, so I just used the path. I would say it was about 50/50.

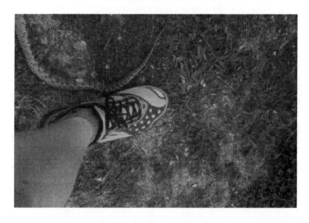

I LOVE these shoes though...I call them ugly in fun. If they keep feeling good, I will probably buy several more pair this year.

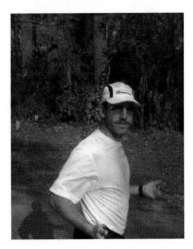

Erik is an interesting fellow, and in fact, a very good runner. The pace we held was definitely more of a challenge for me than him, evidenced by his sprightly form every time we had to move for someone or something. He looked like he could run twice as fast as he was the way he ran. He also has a handlebar mustache...how many of you can say you have run with someone with a handlebar mustache? He is the kind of guy that definitely puts a lot of thought into everyday decisions, and doesn't think in the same box as most of society.

There was a good mix of folks out running, biking, walking, grilling, and you name it this day. We started near the north end of White Rock Lake and by Erik's decision we ran clockwise this day (good choice, I did DFW counterclockwise.) The nice views of the park in my opinion are when you are along either the eastern or western sides of the lake.

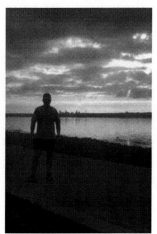

That is Dallas back there...

A habit of mine this last month on my runs is to end up going places I am not "supposed" to go in these parks...nothing different here. On the southern edge of the lake is a dam and a spillway with such a neat pattern in the spillway, that I could resist hopping the "forbidden" fence to take a picture!

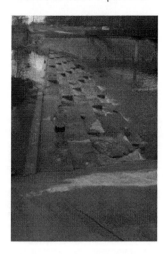

We got some directions from some nice bicyclists when there was a split in the path and headed up the west side of the lake. There were people fishing for croppie, a nice gentleman with a plastic baggie and a grabber thingy picking up trash from along the shore, and just lots of folks enjoying the nice weather in general.

After the run we headed back out, and as we got back on the road, I saw and had to stop for a picture at this hamburger joint. Funny thing is, I don't eat hamburgers anymore, and haven't really drank beer in maybe 9 years...but apparently, this place is for me...

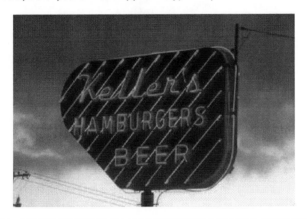

SUNDAY, MARCH 25, 2007

George Bush Intercontinental Airport Run

Got into Houston today, and the wheels in my devious brain starting turning. I was released from duty at around 730pm local and I was ready to go, so I headed out of my hotel and did the circuit around the Houston Intercontinental Airport. Now I have knocked off most of the major Texas airports on my list to run the perimeter. Austin remains...and maybe Fort Worth or El Paso.

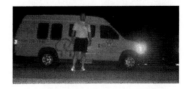

Right off the bat there was a really cool car that I wanted to take a photo of, and then for a long time nothing really interesting presented itself, so I just put my head down and ran.

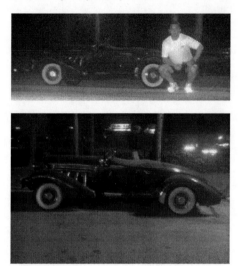

If I am not mistaken this is an Auburn BoatTail. I could have gone up and looked at the emblems, but that would be too easy...

I stopped at gas station on the corner of Lee and Green and got a Gatorade and two dark chocolate candy bars. This was between about 1.5 miles and 2 miles in and I was already sweating pretty good in the humid air, so I think the clerk was wondering what my deal was when I took my stuff and just ran on down the road. I saw a raccoon dart across the road in front of me, but he was too quick to get a photo. Later I also ran by a skunk that had been made into road pizza but I didn't have the stomach to take a photo of that.

I ran by the main entrance to the airport...

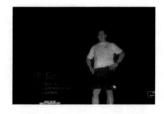

Later on, I found a neat area under the approach lights to one of the runways and took a shot there...

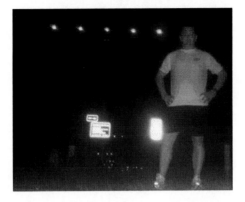

When I got back to Green road with around 1.5 miles to go, two young girls were having trouble getting their car started and I stopped and helped them out. Their starter was going bad and needed smacked...hopefully they change that soon.

I finished my 16.36 miles in 02:45:00 which isn't too bad...if my mental math is right, it works out to right around 10 minutes per mile...which, if I had stopped my watch on all my pee breaks, would probably be a lot better...oh well. I am kind of hoping that when I run the Cleveland marathon in May that I might be able to break 4 hours. That should be right around a 9 minute pace to do so...and that is why I have been checking my watch a little more often lately. I think it will be close. If I prepare well, and rest the few days before the race, I think I have a good shot at it.

MONDAY, MARCH 26, 2007

What happens in Vegas...

I thought I was going to get to run around the Houston airport again tonight, but I was planning to go in the opposite direction. Instead, I got called up for a flight to Las Vegas, and now I am going to run around the Las Vegas McCarran International Airport. I am typing this before I head out...the preliminary distance shows to be about 13.3 miles from my hotel south of the strip. Off I go, the rest will be post run!

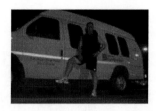

Back at the hotel now, notch up another one for Super Airport Circling Guy. I am such an idiot. I wish I had beautiful trails to run on, but unfortunately when you are a pilot they tend to stick you at hotels next to airports and not state parks. Oh well. Life, lemons, lemonade and all that.

I don't know if it is because I have been a little sick with a cough and stuff, or it is actually the air out here, but after this run I felt like I had breathed in the worst crap of anywhere I else I have ran recently. The post run phlegm party was not what I would prefer.

Well, there is definitely a lot to see when running Vegas, even if you want to hold your breath the whole time. First I passed a sign that made me return back so I could take a picture (I run that fast, by the time my brain processes what I read, I have to turn around and go back...)

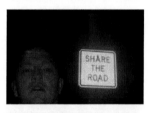

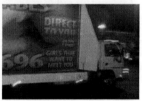

(part of another sign that caught my attention...these billboard vans just circle Vegas all night...I wonder when the girl comes to see you if her car has a little lighted sign on top like the Dominos delivery car?)

My only real goals going down the main Vegas strip were to get a shot of the welcome sign...

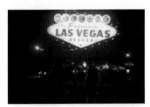

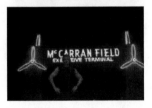

And to try to get a decent shot of the Luxor - the Egyptian casino shaped like a pyramid with the laser beam shooting out it's top...

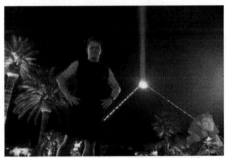

(frickin laser beam....is that so hard?)

I also scored some nice shots at the corner of Tropicana and Las Vegas Blvd (the strip) of both the MGM and New York, New York.

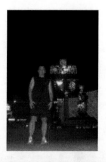

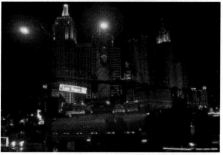

After turning the corner on Tropicana (and shortly after ducking into Atlantic aviation to pee and get a drink of water....) I just put my mind into the running as the next few miles were much less scenic. The next hour passed pretty quickly and before I knew it I was on Sunset Blvd, just hoping for Las Vegas Blvd to get there, so I could make that last left turn and kick for the hotel. It came none to soon, and I ended up getting back to the hotel about 4 minutes longer than planned....I won't say how long, because too many people already assume things about me like I am very concerned about how fast I run....If I wasn't gawking at all the people, the homeless, the party folks, the gamblers, the elderly tourists....etc....I am sure I would have made my time, so big whoop. I had a strong tailwind for the first two legs of the run which really made me feel strong, and then of course had to fight the wind and going slightly uphill over the second half.

This airport thing is really kind of fun, and each time I add a new one to the list, I kind of feel like Rocky Dennis from the movie "The Mask" when he is adding another precious card to his collection of 1955 Brooklyn Dodger cards.

I would continue to have many fun adventure runs in April 2007.

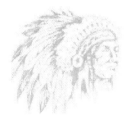

Indian Run April 4th, 2007

After running with Chef Bill Bailey the other day, an idea starting percolating in my devious little brain. We had run by and taken pictures of the Indian statue that stands in Stow, OH near the intersections of Rt. 8 and Rt. 59. I thought of two other Indian Statues in our area and figured it would be interesting to make a run connecting all the statues in our area in one run. After proposing the idea to Bill, he added on a fourth statue that I had forgotten about, and if he complains about the length of this journey I will remind him that his additions took our run from about 11 miles up to the 25 it ended up at.

We agreed to start the run early Wednesday evening so that we could run until we had it all in, without pressure to get done by a certain time, like we would have if we ran the morning like our normal dawn patrol. Bill being the chef extraordinaire and all, I asked him if he wanted to make some Native American flat bread to fuel out efforts (Vince Rucci's idea) and he jumped on it and made us some nice bread with whole grains and oats as well.

Bill also brought us some Indian feathers that he scavenged off of his son's dream catcher and we tied those onto our gear. We had considered doing war paint on our faces, but this never happened. Maybe next year.

61

Unfortunately, the BEAUTFUL weather we have had the last few days in Ohio had to say goodbye for a little while and we started our run in a very light snow and about 35 degree temps. Starting out from Indian number one we made our first turn on Bailey Rd. Very appropriate.

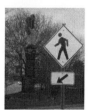

A sign of things to come?

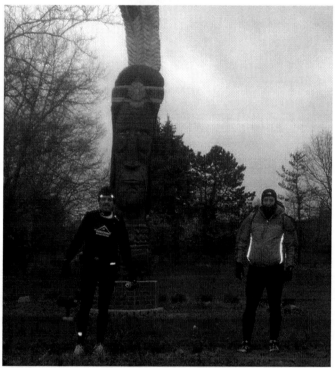

Stow, OH - Rt 59 and Rt 8

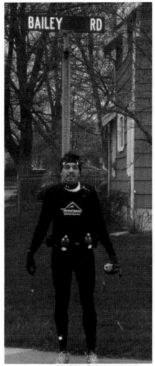

Bailey Rd.

As we approached Truxell Rd headed up State Rd (or old route 8) I realized it would be more fun to run through the Ledges trail between Truxell and Rt 303. We still had daylight so the run through the trail was very pretty. We took one little stop at Ice Box cave and then it was another mile or so until we hit Indian Statue #2 at the entrance to Camp Butler along 303. This statue looks so much like the first one in style that we both thought that maybe it was the same artist.

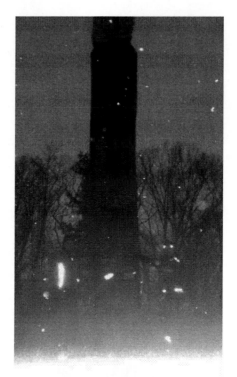

Indian at Camp Butler (Rt 303)

It was at this point, right after the Camp, that I found myself feeling so good nearly halfway in that I almost uttered, "I feel great, and this isn't so bad after all..." Suspicious me clamped my jaws shut and I managed to keep it inside.

We headed down into Peninsula and just past the center of town we picked up the Towpath trail, which would provide us a respite from traffic and noise for a while. By this time it was getting dark and although Bill brought his headlamp, we found we didn't need any light due to the light color of the trail. We decided some point along in here, that we should have Indian names for the run, and Bill came up with Running Blade for him (Chef) and Grounded Eagle for me (Pilot.)

At Bolantz Rd which was several miles down the Towpath we had the good fortune of there being a heated bathroom where we stopped briefly. **Running Blade** was able to fill his waterskin (bottle) and I used the john. Back out onto the trail, it was much more comfortable for us to keep running because of how cold we would get if we slowed down and walked much. My gloves were remarkably wet which made my hands pretty cold. I am not sure if it was sweat that made them so wet, or water that would get out of my bite valve off of my hydration pack when I would use it. A hydration pack is a backpack with a water reservoir built in and a tube and sipping valve that comes over the shoulder for drinking. Mine holds 1.5 liters of water, which seems to be enough for 20 miles in colder weather. I ran out with about 5 miles to go....

When we got to Bath Road along the Towpath we transitioned back to Riverview Road so we would be further away from the infamous "**poop loop**." This is a section of the Towpath trail that goes right by the **Summit County Wastewater treatment plant**. Even from the roadside we got a few pretty good whiffs of everyone's byproducts, but I am sure it was milder than the trailside smell. Along the road **Bill** got out his headlamp and wore it to give the oncoming drivers more warning of our presence.

Once we got to Portage Path road we had another Indian to photo, which is a giant bronze statue of an Indian portaging a canoe. The snow and low light make some of these pictures less than ideal, but that is what we were dealing with so...

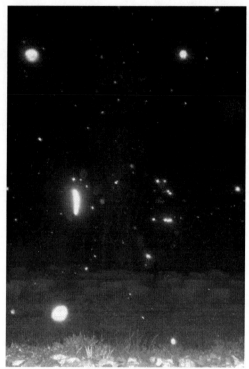

Portaging Indian

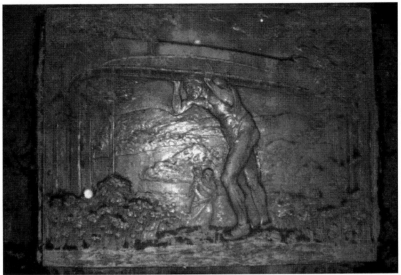

Plaque near the Portaging Indian Statue

Also near the position of the Portaging Indian is a 3 foot tall (or so) Arrowhead that marks that start of the path that the Native Americans would take when portaging their canoes from the Cuyahoga River to the Tuscarawas River 8 miles away. We would pass about 5 more of these arrowhead markers along our way up to Market Street in the last few miles of the run. They are oriented such that each arrowhead points to the next one along the trail. (Do I smell another run cooking up? 8 miles each way - 16 roundtrip to connect them all and return? Bill?)

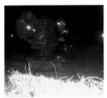

Arrowhead #1

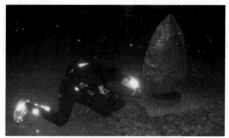
Arrowhead #2

Don't ask me what Bill is doing here, I don't know. I think he was pointing his way along the trail.

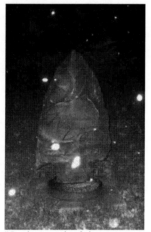
Arrowhead #3, ok enough of these, you get the idea...

Up Portage Path initially is a pretty steep hill, which we committed to walking and then challenged each other into running about 1/4 of it on the way up. Right near the top of this hill you get to pass another local landmark, which is Stan Hywet Hall, a local mansion/castle that was brought over from Europe around the turn of the last century. During this portion Bill is talking about how it was when he ran this stretch during his first marathon, the Akron Road Runner Marathon, which I plan to run next fall.

Just before we got to Market Avenue, we passed **Bailey** avenue, which required a photo with Mr. Bailey of course.... the only bad part is that the name of the road got washed out in the reflection.

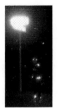

Bailey Avenue

At the point where Portage Path and Market Avenue collide, there was yet another Indian statue. This served as a spot for another picture, and was the place where I called for our ride so when we finished at the last Indian about 2 miles later, we could ride back to the starting point for Bill to get his car.

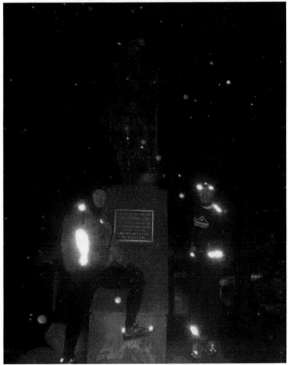

Market and Portage Path

After we turned down Market we were both pretty certain it was all downhill to the finish, well it was elevation wise, but not element wise. We ran maybe a half-mile down Market, and a strong gust front came through with driving winds and snow that cut the visibility down to 1/8 mile or so. The wind was strong enough that I felt like a good gust could knock me down. This didn't last very long, but it did last long enough to do the following to Bill and I...

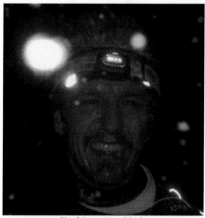

Chef Running Blade

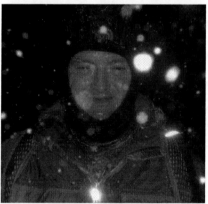

Brave Grounded Eagle

And now, after passing the inclement weather, we had only a mile or so to go, and we got to our last Indian statue at the finish.

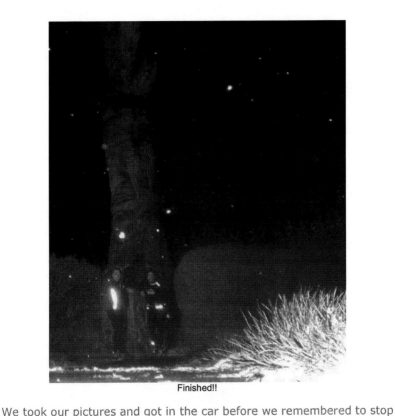
Finished!!

We took our pictures and got in the car before we remembered to stop our watches, which were at 5:09:00 by then, so our best guess is we ran the 25 miles in 5 hours even, and that includes all the stops for photos, peeing, and such. I am very happy with that overall, when I consider it was 1/4 of the distance of a 100-mile race. If I were able to maintain that kind of pace over 100 miles that would be 20 hours, and that would be a dream finish. Of course, I will slow down considerably in the latter stages of a 100, but this should still translate into the ability to finish a 100 miler under the cutoff of 30 hours, and that is the immediate goal for now! I plan on doing this run again, whether it is this summer as another training run, or maybe if we make it a regular run every year, I hope some more folks will join in the trek! Notice below if you click on the photo and zoom in, I put the date of the run on the finisher's "medals" I made.

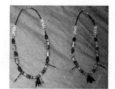

The 2007 finisher's medals!

A note here; The Indian Run is something that Chef Bill and I are now planning on making an annual run during the same week.

Greensboro, NC Airport Run

I got free tonight around 5pm and headed out to circle the Greensboro airport. I had carefully looked on the map and written down the roads where I would have to make all my turns so I wouldn't get lost...

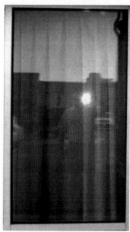

Headed Out

My hotel is about one mile from the airport, so I had to run up S. Regional Road to get there and then start my circle. All was well in the first 3-4 miles as I got warmed up, until I was coming up the road and hit this street sign and knocked it out of the ground with my shoulder...

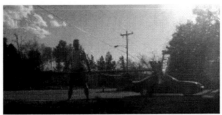

Rippling Street Sign Pulling Muscles

OK, maybe it was just lying there and I wanted to see how heavy it was...

Right at the start of my first wrong turn of the day (first of many) I stopped and took this photo of some clever graffiti...

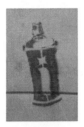

On the return trip backtracking from the dead end I found on my wrong turn journey, I was careful not to run over 14 miles per hour...

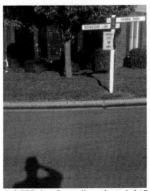

Huh??? Am I reading that right?

What a dead stupid sign and ordinance. I would love to see the transcript of the meeting where some idiots that agreed upon a 14 mile per hour speed limit.

I got back on track and maybe about 4 miles later I was getting all confused again. The road I was supposed to be on ended at a construction site, where it was supposed to go through. I had to choose between going through the construction zone, which was quiet with all the workers gone for the night, or going a few miles down a four lane highway with marginal shoulders...(is that a pun?) I chose the construction site, and for more than half of it, had to walk to avoid losing my shoes in the unpredictable mud.

I got through this area, and after crossing the highway to continue; I was headed back up an off ramp to a normal road, when I found me some road porn. Oh yeah, good old dirty magazine just lying on the road. Two hours later, when I started running again...just kidding. I did take a picture for my friend Tyler Darby (www.aircrewphotos.com) who likes to talk about road porn on his pod cast sometimes. I won't post it here...sorry. There is plenty of porn just a few clicks away for those who are disappointed. If you are online to read this blog, you are not starving for porn.

I decided since I was so much slower than expected with all my wrong turns and trying to figure out what roads were what, that I should stop and eat, so I found a little pizza joint and went in. Got me a small thin crust pizza with cheese and some diet Pepsi. That took a while and was worth the deviation, as their delivery driver gave me some spot on directions for the rest of my run. Without talking to him, I would have easily taken two more wrong turns. Thanks pizza guy!

Well, that is it...got back to my hotel in about double the time I thought it would take. I stopped my watch after the second wrong turn diversion. I won't even try to map it because the roads are so different from what was on Google. I am sure I did somewhere between 15-17 miles.

Burning River Familiarization Run, and then some

Kurt had the good idea that we should turn our normal Sunday run into a familiarization run to see the first 18 miles or so of the Burning River 100 course. Armed with a textual description of the racecourse, we lit out from Squire's Castle at about 8am. Debi and Cindy were committed to stay with us for the first 6 miles and turn back for a total of 12 in their training for the Cleveland half marathon. Josh, Kurt, and I were to continue on the course to the Shadow Lake aid station at mile 18.4 and then back to my car about a mile later.

After a chilly, but not cold, start at the Castle...

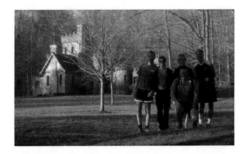

We all headed down the road, warming up quickly from running exertion and spicy banter. Around 5 miles in we started looking for a place for the ladies to take a tinkle with no success and were still looking when they parted paths with us around the 6-mile mark. I suspect they would not pee while still with us for fear that I would sneak a picture of them and post it on here.

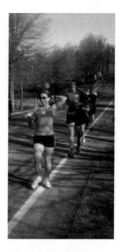

I was noticing that in the first 8 miles or so, I was feeling a little "twinge" on my left knee (again my weaker leg) but also luckily no discomfort from my left hip, which usually squawks a little. In fact, it had felt a little off when running the night before with Josh. Now it was fine. So I babied the knee and kept my footfalls light and quick. Somewhere after 8 miles the knee issue disappeared and I never had another issue. I felt so strong until the finish in terms of body that I was just amazed. May this feeling revisit me on August 4th!

We went South while they went North and we started keeping an eye out for South Woodland road and the Polo Fields park, which would be the second aid station of the race. As we neared it, about a mile out, Josh first recognized the pangs of his hunger from a very limited breakfast of a Luna bar I gave him. We committed to watching for a gas station or store, which we hadn't see in the first 8.5 miles or so...

At the corner before the Polo Fields we knew it was now or never, so we stopped a bicyclist and asked him if he knew of the closest gas station/convenience store. In a fairly thick **German** accent he told us we could go East or West and find a store within about 2.5 miles either way. East seemed best to us, because it was only one road, and there was supposed to be a gas station AND a convenience store. Two miles later while we were looking at nothing but rural road, we were wondering how far his 2.5 miles was going to be.... perhaps in the conversion between kilometers and miles our European friend got confused? After 3 miles I asked a man working on his lawn and he told us the intersection of oasis was .9 miles up the road. 3 dead deer carcasses, a dead raccoon, and precisely .9 miles up the road we were in front of the convenience store.

By now, Kurt and I had also both recognized the pangs of hunger and were more than ready to stuff a few calories down our gullets. I ended up with a Turkey sandwich, a Chicken salad sandwich, a granola bar, a bottle of Mt. Dew (the real deal today to get the extra calories to run on) and a few handfuls of good salty pretzels that Kurt bought. We were all so renewed and starting picking our pace back up as we wandered the 4 miles back to the Polo Fields to enter the Buckeye Trail. We had added 8 miles to our route to find sustenance, and Kurt made the quip that *"Only ultrarunners will run 8 extra miles to find some food!"*

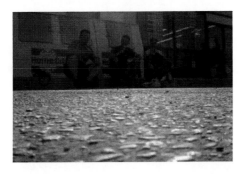

We got to the Polo Fields and after communing with some horse owners and seeing the horses we assessed where the hell the trail was, and after nearly going to wrong way, we headed onto the Buckeye Trail. In here, we recognized the fact that the first 15 miles of the course to this point were mostly flat, and folks were likely to jackrabbit out on race day to a faster start than perhaps they should. I predict just such comments from many race reports after the first race..."I knew I shouldn't start so fast, but it was so flat, and I thought I could bank some miles..."

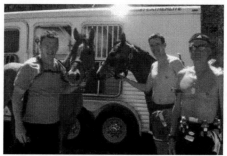
What a bunch of studs!

We counted around 5-6 stream crossings over the next 9 miles and in one of the smaller ones; I looked over and saw a deeper pool just to the left of the crossing. I walked into the pool and it was up to my knees. I stood there for about 40-60 seconds and soaked it in and allowed it to cool my feet, and calves. This turned out to be a very good move as my legs just felt GREAT the last 6 miles or so of our run after that. The biggest issue after we hit the trail was that I ran out of water, even though I refilled at the convenience store, and my mouth was so dry I just couldn't wait to finish and get a drink. With the warmer temps, I had gone through my 1.5 liters of Gatorade I bought, plus a few long drinks of water at the Polo Fields and was just dying for more water through the last 4 miles of our run. So water was my savior and my downfall.... hmmm. On race day there will be three stocked aid stations over this course where I can replenish my water supplies.

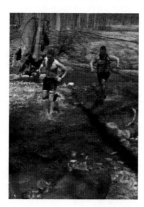

We finished our day with a total of 28.23 miles between the gas station loop, and probably one extra mile on trail as we took a wrong turn and had to wind around and re find our way around Shelterhouse center on the **Bridle Trail**. With our 20k on Saturday morning, my 6.3 miles Saturday night with Josh, and this run I was up to 46.9 miles over the weekend. When I went to the pool Sunday night to try to swim, but couldn't I elected to lift weights instead so I did, and then ran 1.1 miles on the indoor track taking me up to 48 miles with the intention of adding 2 more miles on the road at night to get 50 miles in for the weekend. Sleep, however intervened when I hit my couch at home, and as I write now at 3:40 am, I will not run again. Amazingly to me, my legs are fine, as I feel like I could go out for a 10 miler if I chose, which is good for a guy planning to run 100 miles one day this summer. I will probably go over to the pool this morning though and put in a mile, as I don't have to be available for work until 8 am.

Thanks to Josh for driving up from Cincy! Kurt for planning the run! and Cindy and Debi for providing the "butt beacons" to pull us along the first six miles of our run this morning!

The month of May began with a repeat of one of my absolute FAVORITE adventure runs. I would only be able to do this particular run this spring, and knew I had to enjoy it while the moment lasted...

TUESDAY, MAY 01, 2007

The most important run of my week

This morning I sent an extra lunch with my daughter to preschool, so that when I arrived there at noon, I would be able to sit down and have lunch with her, as well as put her to sleep for naptime after lunch. I have done this once before, last fall, and I knew the distance to be 11 miles, so I set out from my house around 10am to give myself two hours to run over there.

Everything went smoothly, outside of my normal hourly stop to pee on long runs, and I made it to the playground in 1:46:24 (9:40 pace.) I got to play outside for about 15 minutes, answering questions from the shocked student teachers when my daughter told them how I got there, AND where we live.

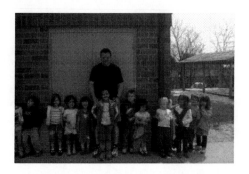

After lunchtime and with naptime starting, I left around 1:15 pm to run home, hoping to get back in time to walk my 10 yr old home from her school. I didn't have a ton of drive to make it because she is used to walking home alone sometimes, and has friends to walk with.... and so when my legs and body weren't enjoying the running, I would just switch to walking on the way back. I walked all the up hills, and even some more on flats.... I would easily say I walked about half the distance coming home, and didn't get back to the house until about 3:40 pm.

I did get two interesting photos on the return trip.... one walking past the starting point of our Indian Run a few weeks back. I noticed how all the walking guys on the sign and intersection light all lined up in front of our Indian statue...here it is.

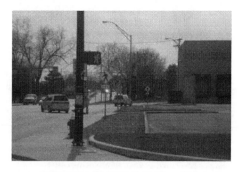

Also, on campus near the art building is some artist's rendition of a giant earthen pot or something.... this was never here when I went to school at Kent.

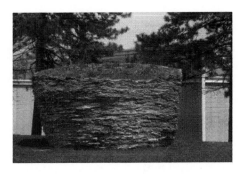

24 hour walk

I have mentioned it a few times in previous posts, but I had this idea a few months back while running with Bob Combs, Jim Harris, and Dave Peterman that to train for running a 100 miler I needed to walk 24 hours. They all endorsed the idea as a productive way to get my psyche ready for the task, so I waited until the weather was acceptable to me to try it. That was yesterday.

I got Kurt Osadchuk on board with the idea and we made plans together to leave Squire's Castle (the starting point of the Burning River 100) at 5am Thursday. 5am because this is the time the race will start on August 4th. With no aid stations in place like race day, a point to point walk like we had planned required a lot of careful planning to make sure we had food and water. We wanted to walk the Burning River course as much as possible for familiarization but the main goal was 24 hours on the feet, so we made some modifications to the plan after 30.3 miles (Station Road) so that we could be re supplied at my car at Boston Store in a reasonable time.

In true college mentality, I was an idiot the night before the walk and didn't go to bed until *2 am* even though I had to leave the house at 3:20 am to drop off supplies and still make the start in time. I swear I did not do this on purpose to add to the difficulty of getting through the walk, but in retrospect now I can look back and say that I did the 24 hours on minimal rest and made it through, so.... Trust me, come race day, I **WILL** have slept 8+ hours the night before.

With all the supplies positioned, we arrived at Squire's Castle and started the walk at exactly 5am. We got there like one minute early, stepped out of the car and started walking; it could not have been timed better. We had a beautiful clear sky under a full moon and temps at the start of the walk were 49 degrees or so, and any *runner* knows that this is practically balmy to us right? Remember I said we were WALKING for 24 hours? We were miserable and cold the first 2+ hours of the walk because we had dressed like we would have dressed for running and until the sun came up we were cold. Walking just doesn't generate the body heat that running does... Believe it or not, between the cold temps and lack of sleep the first two hours or so of the day were probably the hardest for me. Not that I wasn't sore and tired of walking by hours 22 - 24, but those first two hours were the only time I really considered whether I would be happier coming back another day.

Right around 4 miles in, at about 6:15 am, I saw an electrical box on a telephone pole with a warning that the cover could be hot...so naturally, all cold and miserable I tried to go bask in some of it's heat. Talk about false advertising, this thing was as cold as we were!

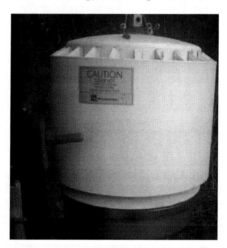

Having run this route just a few weeks back I knew there were some areas coming up which should allow the newly rising sun to strike us quicker than where we were. For a long time, although the sun was up hillsides on the left (east) side of us were blocking it and keeping us in the shade. By the time we were within a few miles of the Polo Fields we were regularly in the sunshine and starting to thaw out.

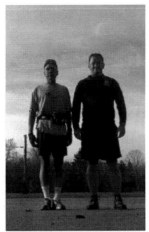
Kurt and I at the Polo Fields

Out of the Polo Fields we were onto the Buckeye Trail and I am already starting to think about the point several miles ahead of us where we took a wrong turn while running the trail a few weeks back. It is at the intersection of Chagrin River Rd. and Miles Road, where we had previously scoped out and taken the wrong trail for several miles. We stopped and looked everywhere we could think of until just around the corner, where we hadn't looked last time, we found the actual Buckeye Trail with its blue blaze marking. These issues will not be present on race day because of the folks marking the course, but when you are trying to follow it alone, it can be very easy to miss these turns.

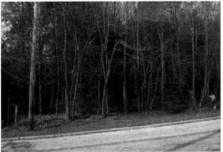
Which way did he go? (the spot where Kurt is pointing is the real Buckeye Trail)

After we progressed along the BT and shortly before we arrived at what would be the next aid station on the race, we hit one of my favorite streams. This is where there is a spot about 2 feet deep where I can soak my legs in cold water and relieve some of the fatigue that has set in to this point. It really works, like icing tired muscles after a hard workout.

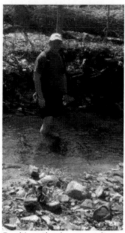
Soaking the leg muscles...

At Harper Ridge aid station we just stayed on the trail, although I did sit down in the grass and take a few minutes to clear out some debris from my shoes and socks, as well as reapply some more bodyglide to my feet to make sure the blisters didn't come. After about 10 miles, I had a feeling the rest of the day that I guess some would call a "hot spot" on the bottom of my feet, but it never developed into a blister...I just keep reapplying the glide, and it was fine. I also would change socks and shoes later, when the night came. Another word about shoes; I was wearing my favorite Brooks Cascadia kermit green kickers, which never before had a problem with pebbles or grit getting into them when I ran in them. Walking seems to be different though, because I was emptying my shoes every few miles today.... until I tried something. I moved the laces at the top of the shoe to the very furthest back eyelet along my ankle, which would be a bother when running, causing the shoe to rub me raw on my ankle. While walking I didn't get rubbed though, and it kept the shoe tighter back there and kept out a lot more grit.

Just after Harper Ridge we were anticipating the lunch stop, which would occur near the Shadow Lake aid station, where Kurt's mom lives just a half mile off of the course. We called her, and she was gracious enough to go to McDonalds and get us grub. Now, McDonalds is somewhere I do NOT eat, but today would be an excepting since we were expending so many calories. I got three grilled chicken sandwiches with mustard instead of mayo, and Kurt got three large french fries. We took about 15 minutes to sit and eat this instead of trying to carry it with us as we went.

After this we were back onto wooded Buckeye Trail as we headed for the Egbert aid station and the Bedford Reservation. We wound around and around along Tinker's creek and were presented with many wild creatures. The deer in here are very tame and let me get to within 15 feet at times. There were also geese, snakes, great blue herons, red-tailed hawks, etc.

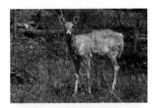

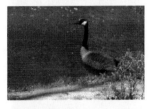

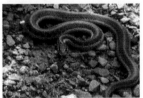

This last guy wasn't sitting on the trail, but made the mistake of making noise in the leaves as I walked by, so I got a stick and pulled him out on the trail for a photo op. We couldn't decide if he was the harmless gardener snake or what, so I just handled him with a stick.

Out of Egbert aid station, the Buckeye Trail has a spur which goes down to Tinker's Creek but is not part of the race.... we took it. It was not intentional, and we backtracked once to check we were on the trail, but made it all the way down to the creek before realizing there were no more BT blazes and I got out the map. We saw that we had to go back up to Egbert and head out on the correct portion of the trail to stay on the racecourse. Before we left the creek however, I took of my shoes and soaked the legs again for about 2 minutes. Every time I did this, my legs felt much fresher for the next few hours.

Through the reservation the trail crosses and re crosses the Gorge Parkway several times and we were looking forward to the Alexander Road aid station as an indicator we were making progress, and then on to the Station Road aid station where Kurt had his car parked at 30.3 miles and we had drinks and food in the trunk in coolers. We made steady progress and got into Station Road at around 7pm.

Along the towpath trail leading up to Station Road, I had the urge for about the 100th time this day, and waited for a moment where no one was in sight so I could pee. Well, of course, a biker comes around the bend, but seeing it is a guy, I just keep peeing into the weeds. This is about a mile before Station Road, and this goomba felt it important to assert that there was a bathroom just ahead, with a touch of disdain in his voice, as if I should be embarrassed to be peeing in the weeds. I simply said "Oh thank so much buddy! You are a big help!" but what I **wanted** to say was much worse.

Kurt had called his wife and asked her to meet us here so that he could say goodnight to his daughter and I chimed in asking if she could bring some fig newtons. Ever since Tanya had some when we were running the Mohican course a little over a month ago, and she shared them with me...I have been eating those things like they are crack cocaine. They taste so damn good to me, and they even make a whole grain version now. Kurt's wife showed up with the goods and I got my fix, and Kurt got his fix, and after a short time at the coolers to refill our water bottles etc., we were back underway.

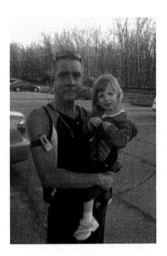

After Station Road is where we made the decision to forgo the actual racecourse and just walk straight down the towpath to Boston Store for several reasons. This would allow me to see my kids before their bedtime, and also to get some more food and drinks from my car, which was there. Then we would have my car as a base of operations the rest of the night. We planned on doing the Pine Lane trail, as well as the Brandywine loop once each and then see where we were before time was up in terms of where to go.

Station Road is only about 4.5 miles or so from Boston Store, so we made good time, and got a bathroom break, each had a 6 inch sub from subway, and after a little stretching, got back underway. Now back in the darkness as the sun had set while we approached Boston Store, we wore our headlamps and headed up into the woods. I was excited to see the portion of the trail that was falling away after the earthquake of several weeks ago, and it did not disappoint. There is this HUGE, make that HUGE! section of trail that is falling away from the rest of the hillside, and is clearly being held up pretty much only by the roots of trees growing there. If I had to guess, I would say the amount of dirt in the piece falling away would FILL 3-4 dump trucks. It is impressive to see, and is even splitting a growing tree from the roots up through the middle. I wish I had a photo, but since it was getting dark, and I was tired of carrying my backpack, I left the camera and just about everything in the car over those last loops.

We gave the unstable portion of trail a VERY wide berth and got back moving. Somewhere along the trail about three miles in we are

walking and out of nowhere we hear a coyote howling maybe a half
mile (wild guess) off to our right.... shortly followed by a different
answering coyote a similar distance off to our left. I am not saying this
didn't bother me, because it was spooky, but it FREAKED Kurt out! The
decision was not in question; there was no way he was coming back
via this trail.

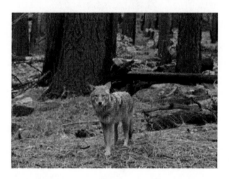

When we got to the end of the trail, we turned right down Rt. 303 and
walked into Peninsula. We went to Lock 29 so we could both go to the
bathroom, and get some water refills. We took about 5 minutes there
while we decided whether to go back up the towpath to Boston Store,
or to head up 303 to Riverview Rd. and down that way.

We ended up going via the roads, which actually had me pretty tense
and freaked out, because there is a medium sized dog at one of the
houses along Riverview Rd, which has chased us running by there
before and come right out to the road where we were, as if there were
no invisible fence or anything. The last time through there I was in a
group of 7-8 runners, but tonight with just the two of us, I worried
that he would have the nerve to actually attack. I found a nice sturdy
stick, and also a hefty rock to deter him if necessary. My apprehension
was undeserved however because we walked right past all those
houses and only saw a few more deer.

Back into Boston Store, another bathroom break for Kurt...grab a few
more fig newtons, etc...and we figured we would have the time to walk
most of the Brandywine trail. At this point we weren't trying to walk
fast.... just walk...the goal of time on feet was all that mattered, so we
just lazily walked along with no urgency.... We left Boston Store at
2:28 and figured we had 2:32 left, so we had 1:16 to walk, then turn
around and walk back...even if we didn't finish the Brandywine loop.
We got going, and were feeling pretty good.... I was most hopeful that

we would get to the stream crossing on Brandywine because that is one of my most favorite places in the woods...and we did.

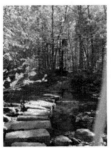

One of my favorites

It was crossable mainly because someone placed some extra rocks on the larger ones you normally crossed on. The large rocks were mostly submerged and would have required wet feet...After we crossed we both decided we had enough time to do the whole loop. The funny thing we realized in here was that while walking we were probably going faster uphill than downhill, because we could just power uphill, but going downhill we were taking very careful steps so as not to fall, or twist an ankle or something.

On the way back downhill on the return side of Brandywine, I learned something I will try to remember.... I decided what it would feel like to run a little during the 24th hour of my day, and I ran the downhill portions a little. Amazingly, running them was easier on my knees and muscles than the walking was at this point. I think it is going to be an exercise of seeing when I can run, and when I can walk during the 100 milers. Kurt and I have talked a lot about how deceptive the first 20 miles of this race are to folks who haven't seen the southern half of the course. You may be tricked into thinking it is a relatively flat 100 until you get into the Cuyahoga Valley.... and then look out quads!

We actually got back to the Boston Store at 04:46 am from the Brandywine Loop so we walked out again on the towpath for 7 minutes, turned around and walked back to bring us to exactly 5am, 24 hours after our little journey began.

I learned a lot of little things about myself this journey, like that I want to stash many extra socks in drop bags during the race, I want to work on finding a better compression short for me, because my thighs and nether areas chafed way too much.... I was happy with the eating

I did, and the energy levels I had through they day, but also recognize that I will need more overall calories on race day, because my energy will be used quicker due to running vs. walking.

I come away with the one main thing I was hoping to come away with...I HAVE NOW BEEN ON THE RACE COURSE FOR 24 HOURS STRAIGHT AND I KNOW I CAN DO IT!!!!I just have to run a little more of the race come August.... oh, and I also get another 6 hours on race day to finish.... We did an estimated 51 miles this day, although I will try to map it and pin down a more accurate distance including any wrong turns, and detours for food, etc.

So the day for the big marathon had come, and I was very excited to get going...though I had been running for quite some time now, I still had a lot to learn...Cleveland's streets would be my tutor this time around...

SUNDAY, MAY 20, 2007

30th Annual Cleveland Marathon
A Personal Best and a missed goal.

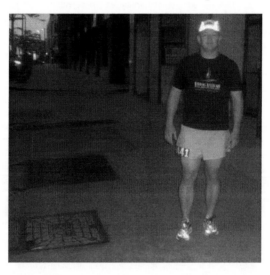

Cindy apparently, re-sublaxeted her cuboid, so I will have to be watching carefully on her blog for the full report. That is still a pretty good time to have fought through an injury. I never saw Kurt or Maria today, although I had my eyes peeled. It took me 17 miles to find Roger and then (if you can't tell we ended up finishing together...photo later in this post.)

I had made plans on making an attempt on my first 4 hour marathon (or just under) and today was the day to go for it. I got a bib as part of the 4:00 pace group and lined up and started the race with them. Standing in line I chatted with a few other 4 hour hopefuls...one a young lady (cute as hell) named Jeremie (yes Jeremie, I asked) and another fellow on his third marathon like me. Soon, I saw Cindy and moved up to start near her...she was aligned with the 3:50 pace group hoping to run a 1:55 half marathon herself. I didn't see much harm in starting with them, as early pace in marathons is more determined by crowds than by what you want to do usually.

Cindy and I stayed near each other for most of the first 3 miles, and when she slowed a bit and moved to the center of the road on Rt. 2 near Edgewater trying to get a glimpse of and give a shout out to Tony, I kept going and never saw her again until the finish line. I stayed in between the 3:50 and 4:00 pace group for the first 15 or so miles....sliding back and forth as I took my three stops to pee on the side. I just wasn't ready to go out of my shorts like SOME quicker runners I know do...I was afraid of getting some in my socks or something, and I don't think my race is determined by small factors like that yet. I am still in the phase of marathoning where conditioning is the biggest determining factor and small variances aren't as big of a deal. What I will say though is that it gets a little harder to get up to pace each time after stopping though.

Coming back from the West side of Cleveland around 8 miles or so, I started to notice that not wearing compression shorts under my sexy green running shorts was a stupid mistake. I was getting an irritating case of "chub rub" where the thighs rub each other and chafe. I could tell that without something to help, this would be bleeding and painful by mile 26.2. I formulated a quick plan.... my support crew were all supposed to try to see me by Jacob's field for a halfway photo. I knew that they would probably still be carrying my backpack, which had bodyglide and blister shield in it. I would rub on some bodyglide and then dash it with the powder of blister shield as well to try to ease the rub and pain. They WERE there! Thank you! I stopped...rubbed.... dashed.... and got two kisses from my daughters as I headed out, with the wife yelling...no kisses! Get moving! HaHa...taskmaster.... she shot these photos.

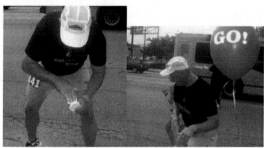

I love the juxtaposition of the balloon with the "GO!" printed on it, and the clean air bus in the background.

The last time I peed it took me several miles to reel in the 4:00 group and I stayed with them for several more miles until somewhere around mile 19 or so. Roger and I had found each other, but were both kind of tired and elected to sprinkle in a few walks on some small hills. After the first few walks we were still on pace to just make our 4:00 goal, but somewhere around mile 21-22 we both saw the hopes dissipate. We were running in sight of each other, trading the "lead", but we weren't holding the 9:09 pace necessary to stay on track anymore. I think we were much closer to 10:00.

A note here of thanks; at around mile 22 or so, I came up a short rise (running thankfully! not walking) and I hear a familiar voice say, "Mike!" It was Vince Rucci of Vertical Runner (www.verticalrunner.com) in Hudson, OH. He had a pack with him and the next words out of his mouth (after I pointed to my VR hat) were, "Do you need anything?" I was well hydrated and fed, so I quipped back as I passed him "how about some cocaine or amphetamines?" Then, I was out of earshot and gone.... the moment however stayed with me for two reasons over the next mile or so. First of all, I am always so impressed by Vince, Mel, and Steve of Vertical Runner. They put me at ease and are always so helpful in all matters running...whether it is gear selection or even training or racing advice. The second reason the moment stuck with me is that instead of asking for illegal narcotics, I thought in the next 20 minutes, I should have asked for a free pair of shoes...or even a big discount! Vince - you reading this?

When Roger and I really realized that our dreams of a 4-hour marathon had slipped away was at the 23-mile mark. With just over a 5k to go we were looking at about 26 minutes to run it and break 4 hours. A 26 minute 5k on the hilly course remaining would have been decent if we were rested...but didn't seem possible with the miles already on our legs. We talked briefly about it and decided rather than push hard for a 4:05 or something we would ease up and cruise in to whatever happened. Obviously what happened from above was a 4:12:11, which is a PR for me by about 7 minutes over me previous best 4:19.

The best part of the finish was that my wife allowed my daughters and their cousin to come out and run across the finish line with me. Normally that is a big no-no at races for them, but I guess she had seen enough other kids doing it that she relented.

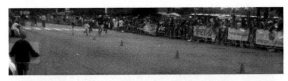

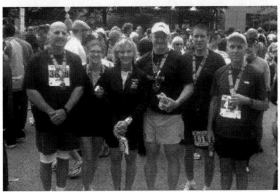

I have no issues with my failure to break 4 hours, although it would have been precious to me to repay the confidence my neighbor Tony has had in me these past two weeks. I know that I did not do enough marathon specific training, as I basically like to do long runs all the time, and never push the speed enough. In the future I will do a marathon training plan for the 4-6 weeks preceding my next marathon and see how I can do then. I also think I have been carrying some extra weight around, because I have not been monitoring my calories as carefully as I used to, and haven't been hitting the scale lately. That much will be changing starting now. I am going to weigh in tonight, and set a new two-month goal for a weight that I want to run Burning River at!

I may add to this blog post if I recall any other items of interest...or if I can get any juicy pictures from fellow runners, or the web. I did see one guy fall out near the end and need medical...as well as someone throwing up right after the finish line.... yummy.

The marathon behind me now, it was time to start getting serious about training for the Burning River 100! June came upon the land of Ohio, and with it my opportunity to experience my first 100 mile race. I would volunteer first as a trail marker, then an aid station volunteer and finally to pace for the Trail Goddess Kim...but first, I had to take a crack at Another Dam 50k to try to finish one...literally.

SUNDAY, JUNE 03, 2007

So Dam Hot! Another Dam 50k

Englewood Metropark near Dayton, OH
June 2, 2007

While I was home this week, I was going to take revenge on my 50k from January when I chose to quit after the marathon distance. I was going to go to the same Buckeye Trail course and run it now. When I started asking around for anyone who wanted to join me, Josh suggested instead that I come down and run Another Dam 50k with him. I accepted.

Because I did not want to stay overnight down there, I had to leave at about 3:30am from my house to drive down to the race. It started at 8 am and I got there at about 6:45 to register. I was the first raceday registration and I got number 50, appropriate for my first 50k finish! After registering I milled around helping the volunteers move coolers and stuff to the aid station. When I went back to my car at 7:15 there was a message from Josh that he had overslept and wasn't coming to the race. Damn! I left my mp3 player at home because I was running with a friend.

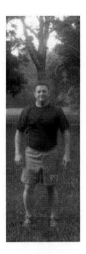

Shortly after that Josh called and said that he wanted to still come and just start late. COOL! So we agreed that I would go ahead and run the first 4.4 mile loop and then look for Josh because that would be about the time he should show up.

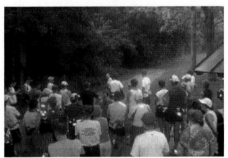

Pre race briefing about one minute prior to start.
For those racers who show up on time!

So I ran the first loop in :44 and when I got back as I was filling my water bottle, Josh showed. I had pre-registered him and all he had to do was sign the paper and head out.

We headed out together on the 3.5 mile shorter loop, which was almost entirely in the shade of the forest, so that meant at the end of my race, Josh would have to run a 4.4 mile loop to complete his 50k.

It had been Josh who proclaimed that we were going to run a very slow 50k because he is getting close to the Mohican 100 race June 16. He said he wanted to do a 16 minute or so mile pace, for a total of around 8:30 for the 50k. I was fine with this, my main goal was just to finish a 50k and get more training miles in.

Well, first let me tell you, that for me at least running a 16-minute mile is not feasible. It is harder to slow down to that type of shuffling pace. I need to run some, walk some if I want to do 16-minute miles. Well, every time we walked for any significant time, we agreed that running felt better (especially later in the race) so we ended up just discarding this 16-minute mile thing and doing what we could. Honestly, our overall pace this day was just about what it would have been if I were racing the race for time. Our pace per mile based on my finishing time was 12:24. This includes all the time spent at the aid station between loops, which was a good amount, as we really didn't hurry like we would in a race situation.

In fact, at the aid stations, I changed shoes twice, once even changing the insoles in one pair, to a set of **gel insoles** that I had frozen to see if the cooler temps would help the feet/overall feeling. The insoles had not stayed THAT cold in my little cooler with ice, so there was not much effect. I also spent about 5 minutes on one stop holding two frozen **gel packs** in my crotch, and a bag of frozen veggies (**peas**/corn) under each armpit, to help cool me down. This felt good, but it is hard to tell if there was much effect there either. Because there were no real stream crossings, I never got a chance to do the thing where I soak my legs to make them feel better.

We kept up a pretty constant pace through the race, slowing slightly, but in general we walked the same hills every time, and only sprinkled in a few small walk breaks at random spots. Again, most times if felt better just to keep running. I look forward to seeing the time splits if they publish them to see how much we slowed each lap. I did something here that I did at the Cleveland marathon. I left my watch in the car. I noticed somewhere around 23 miles in that I was already *fantasizing* about how good it was going to feel to lay down in the **grass** and **shade** and relax while Josh ran his last loop.

Before the last loop, I arranged a volunteer to hold my camera and take some photos of us when we can out of the woods the last time.

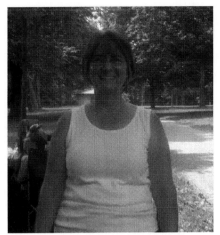

Marna

Her name was Marna and the plan was that as we neared the edge of
the woods, I would shout a loud "Hooo-de-hooo" and she would know
to be ready. This had Josh cracking up as I did it very loudly three
times. Marna heard us coming and got these shots (thank you Marna!)

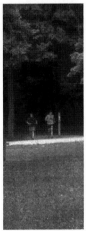

hooo-de-hooo

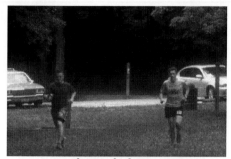

hooo-de-hooo

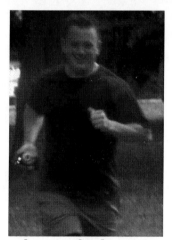

hooo-de-hooo!

During the race, we noticed that we were leapfrogging with one lady named Ingrid and a man named Al, who I came to calling the dirty old man, because about halfway through the race he tripped on a root and rolled across his back covering it in dirt. He was fine though.

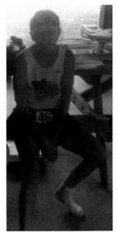

Ingrid

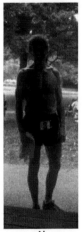

Al

Ingrid was the champion of getting through the aid station fast and we watched her closely. We weren't trying to hurry the aid station visits because our mindset was not to race per se, but we knew we could learn from her for real race days when we wanted to do a good time. She came into the aid station slightly behind us every time, and left before us **every** time.

Another funny thing about Ingrid was that during the first loop without

Josh I was running behind her for some time near the dam, and I noticed that she brings her feet up kind of high behind her when she runs. Stupid me thought about saying something to her about her stride and this being a waste of energy....I maintained self control and kept my dam(n) mouth shut....well 5 minutes later as we are running across the face of the dam we are side by side and chatting when she tells me about the 5 100 mile races she has finished, etc....and I realize how dam(n) stupid I would have been to offer her running advice. She really was strong runner (she is 58) and was a motivation for me all day, thinking of if I will be able to run like that at 58.

I finished in 6:32:33. The results page shows splits of 1:24:22 (7.9 miles), 2:53:08 (15.8 miles), 4:41:39 (23.7 miles), and the finish of 6:32:33 for 31.6 miles. Another way of looking at it is that the loops took:
1st loop - 1:24:22
2nd loop - 1:28:46
3rd loop - 1:48:31
4th loop - 1:51:54

Here the loops I mention are the 3.5 and 4.4 combined, or 7.9 miles each. The course was 4 circuits of the 7.9 mile loop which itself was divided into the 3.5 and 4.4 mile distance loops.

Josh officialy got a 7:12:21 finishing time, but he was only really running about 6 hours 26 minutes, because of showing up late.

This is obviously a PR for me, because it is the first 50k I have finished. This was a very nice race to run, and on a day with 70-degree temps it would be an absolute ideal race setting. There were very few hills, and the only section that was kind of a pain in the ass was the mile or so running across the dam, and that was just due to the heat. The temps today were around 90 degrees in the sun. It was probably 10 degrees hotter on the dam than in the woods. I was running out of **water** by the end of the 4.4 mile dam loop every time due to the heat. I took about 9 S! caps during the race (electrolyte capsules - basically salt, etc.) These are taken to replace the salt and minerals you lose during sweating, and if not taken, a runner will cramp up excessively and usually have a hard time continuing. In fact, we ran into one runner who had a severe hamstring cramp and once he took some caps he recovered and ran the rest of the day.

Josh finished his last loop faster than I ran the first so in reality his time running the 50k distance was between 4-6 minutes faster than mine, but in the results of the race it will show that I was faster than him, because I started on time. I will take it. It will probably be the only time I ever beat Josh in a race! Thanks Josh for the invite, and for getting your ass out of bed and coming even if late!

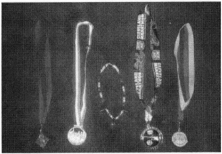

My current medal collection: Towpath half, NYC marathon, Indian 25, Cleveland marathon, Another Dam 50k.

Now, I get to go do some 100 mile volunteering and pacing...

MONDAY, JUNE 18, 2007
Mohican 100 Trail Race

My experience this weekend began with arriving on Friday afternoon to the campground at the start/finish line of the race around 4pm. There was a pasta dinner about to begin and after finding our way to the cabin we would share with Kim (and watching 72 year old Leo flirt with my wife - with his furry chest of white hair blowing in the breeze...), we spent some time at the race pavillion chatting with different runners and friends. I spent some time with Vince of Vertical Runner and met many new friends, awaited Josh, reviewed race day strategy with Kim, as well as aid station duties with Vince.

Once the spaghetti and side salad was consumed, I found out Vince was planning a run of the **Blue Loop** and I invited myself along. I would not get to run the **Blue Loop** with Kim in the race and wanted to see it so bad. Vince and his pups Sadie and Dexter, Mike George, my wife, and I all headed over to the **Blue Loop** around the time that all the runners were getting their pre-race briefing. I cleared it with Kim before I went, because I did not want her worried in any way that it would affect my pacing ability for her the following night. She said

GO!

My wife is not a runner (yet) so the **loop** would be run by Vince (w/pups), Mike, and I. I enjoyed this quite a bit, and had really looked forward to seeing the hand over hand climb at Little Lyon Falls that I had so often read about. It was really neat, and Vince's dogs made it up as well...Sadie climbed and Dexter needed a little push from the cheetah, during which I think he clawed Vince up. My wife stayed behind and enjoyed the area near the Covered Bridge (henceforth CB - a central point of the race.)

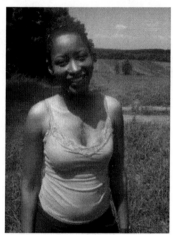

Beautiful Wife

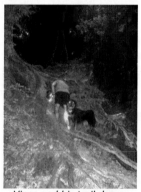

Vince and his trail dawgs

We never had a final time elapsed for running the **blue loop** because Mike stopped his watch accidentally, but we were all good and sweaty when we were done, so we know we did a good job. After going back to the Campground, my wife and I drove a little ways back towards town to find some more food, and also some cell phone signal to say goodnight to the kids who were staying with my parents.

Got to bed fairly early for us, and I would wake up with Kim so I could witness the start of the race, something I did not want to miss. Kim and I got her last bits of running gear ready and after her ceremonial prerace poop for her (sorry Kim, but real life is real life) we headed to the start around 4:30am. I was able to shake hands and wish good luck to Kim, Josh, **Roy** (going for #10 and the 1000 mile buckle), and many others I have come to know.

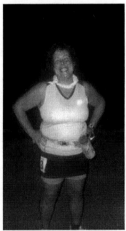

The Trail Goddess beams as she awaits the starting horn!

The race packet says they start the race PROMPTLY at 5:00 no matter what. Bullshit. They were still trying to check everyone in at this time and didn't start the runners til around 5:07 by my watch.
Off they went, and off I went, back to the sleeping bag for another hour or so of slumber. We got up and went into town to get some breakfast before we would have to report to Hickory Ridge aid station for our duties starting around 8:30am.

As we awaited the leader of the race, we stocked our aid station up with water, Gatorade, GU2O, fruit, pretzels, fig newtons (!!!), raisins, peanut butter and jelly sandwiches, various candies, and a few first aid type items and a body lube called Chamous Butt'R that I had never seen before, but later used to lube my feet before pacing.

Aid station work is pretty straight forward. You fill their water bottles, and basically do whatever you can to get them what they need quickly, so they can get their asses back down the trail. Good aid stations mottos:

"Take whatever you need, and get the hell outta here!"

"Beware the chair" (courtesy of Roy Heger to me last winter)

"Drop from the race? Why don't you just sit over there and think about that for awhile....we can't get you a ride right now anyways..." (courtesy of Vince Rucci, saved a guy's race....he stayed with us over an hour...left and went on to finish in 21:30....afterwards he was so grateful to Vince!)

You know I had the camera ready awaiting everyone's arrivals. Here are a FEW of my friends coming in:

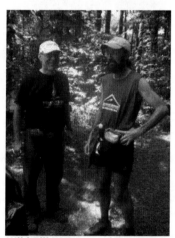

Wild Bill Wagner and **Roy Heger**

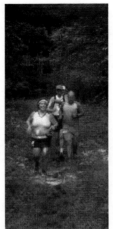

Kim! (aka Trail Goddess - look at her worshippers!)

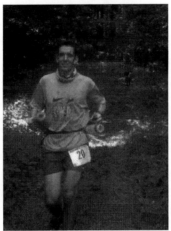

Josh (mile 25 of his first 100 miler - just three marathons to go....)

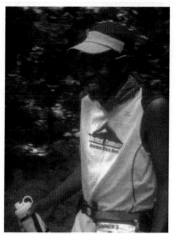

Fred Davis! (he ran 500 miles in 10 days about a month ago...)

Our aid station would be at miles 25.8 and 68.0 during the race. I would actually go through here as a pacer later on with **Kim**. We closed down the aid station for two hours around lunchtime, because all the runners were through for the first time, and the leaders would not be back through until late afternoon. On our way out to lunch in town, fate brings me to the intersection of Rt. 3 and Rt. 97 at the same time as guess who...

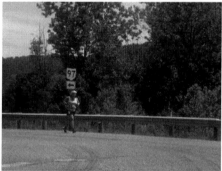

*Here is **Kim** midway through her first **Orange Loop**, a spot we would run together about 13 -14 hours later at night.*

Back at the aid station in the second shift the runners would be more spread out and we would watch the lead change as the first runner who came in had to sit awhile and one or two guys passed him while he was there. The first female runner came through in about 4th place overall: Connie Gardner, no surprise to anyone around here, she is legendary. The second female was a surprise though, Cristal Harris I think, and it was her FIRST ultra of any kind. Only marathons before (are you listening Tony!) She stayed in second place (female 2nd, they talk about it that way) and finished her first 100 miler there, maybe you can contact her Tony and get some strategy? **Red**, can we expect to see you out there soon? You can do it!

I was happy to be able to see **Roy** come through the second time around before I had to head out to the Fire Tower (mile 60.9 on the **Green Loop**) to await Kim to pace her. The comments to **Roy** from Vince and Joe Jurczyk when he came through were "968 miles done, only 32 to go...." This was referring to his 10th finish or 1000 miles.

When I got to the Fire Tower I reconnected with Wendy from the February training run and she was awaiting her husband Rich who was somewhere near Kim. SHE is the evil being behind my fig addiction. Back in Feb when I was out of food and we had a few miles to go on our 25 or so mile run, she offered up the fig and I bit...now I need to find a place specializing in Fig Rehab because of her. Fig Pusher! She has two very polite teenagers and we talked for a while waiting on Kim and Rich. At some point, I overheard a young looking guy in front of me talking about being signed up to run his first 100 miler in August. I approached him and his name was Christian from Columbus and he was 27. We talked a lot about the BR course and eventually when he talked about needing more trail and night running experience, I asked him why not run with Kim and I? I knew she wouldn't mind. So he says sure, he wanted to run about 10 miles and he will run out with us awhile and then come back.

We move out and the first leg is only 2.5 miles down to the CB. Things are going well, Kim is looking so DAMN STRONG! I marvel at how she is running when I remember how I felt after my first 50 miler. As we near the CB she tells me to run ahead and ask the podiatrists located there to be ready to repair two blisters on the sides of her heels. (Kim, let me know if you think those are because of shoe choice? sock choice?) I do so, and they get ready while I go fill water bottles and get Kim and I some soup and stuff. She gets there and they start fixing the feet and my duties included getting her finishing bag (normally called a "drop bag" by everyone else, but I got to be me....) and bringing it back so she can get what she needs. As I watched the doctors work, I wondered to myself why one of the spare doctors couldn't do the left ankle/heel while the first one worked on the right?

I am an idiot, why didn't I speak up? After about 10-12 minutes the other doctor suggests this and I whip off Kim's shoe, bandage, and sock so the doc can get to cutting. (Worshipping at the foot of the trail goddess here.)

Think about that though, that is maybe 12 minutes of WASTED time letting the docs do one foot only, and I am supposed to be her helper.... just standing there with my mouth shut! I reiterate... I am an IDIOT.

When Kim got to me at Fire Tower she had just under one hour of cushion time on the cutoff there, and when we left at CB, I could see that we would have very little cushion at all at the next stop of Hickory Ridge (mile 68.0) I was excited crossing the bridge and going into the woods, because I had not run any of the Orange Loop at all. It is primarily uphill to Hickory Ridge so of course we mixed in a good amount of walking with a still impressive amount of running to me for this late in the race. As we got closer and closer to HR I was more worried about the cutoff, and hatched the plan that I would take the water bottles ahead and fill them while Kim either stopped VERY briefly or not at all depending on her needs. I charged into the aid station hard and as I was filling them and grabbing stuff, she just ran right on through and kept going. So I blasted out and took her the bottles, almost forgetting my camera and her Ipod.

Well, by now we had suckered Christian into running the whole night with us because he had no headlamp of his own and we suggested it would be dangerous to run back alone in the dark. He was an easy sell though, because he recognized the value of the experience he was getting for August's race. He borrowed Kim's extra light and ending up running with us all night. We were treated to stories about his gay alter ego that he keeps on Myspace and that kept us laughing all night.

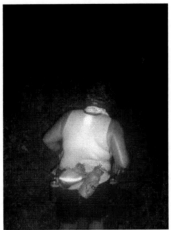

*Here is **Kim** running the **Orange Loop** towards Grist Mill.*

We wound around and around down the **Orange Loop** towards Grist Mill and I had gotten the cutoff time back at Hickory Ridge so I could plan our attack. They said 3:23 am and at the halfway point down Hickory Ridge, it was going to be too damn close for comfort. I began cracking the whip and doing everything I could think of to get **Kim** to run faster. I made jokes to take her mind off the pain in her legs, I ran ahead and while Christian talked to her, I kept the pace up hoping she would follow and go faster just trying to stay close to me...At the end of the loop coming off the last hill, I could see it was just crazy close, and I started really pushing her verbally by telling her that she had better make sure I was getting **everything** she had short of injury.... telling her that her race was RIGHT NOW.... telling her a story I heard about how we can do more than we think when we are fatigued like this. Keep in mind that this is 3am and she has been running since 5am.... 22 hours. Dammit if **Kim** didn't push herself and just put her head down and make that cutoff! We got in and they informed me the cutoff was actually 3:35 and we had 5 minutes to spare.

This is where one of the funniest things happened. **Kim** told me she needed my light because her batteries were weak and I rushed it to her as she went along side this building at the Grist Mill that I ASSUMED was a bathroom. After a few minutes, and knowing that we had no time to spare I was asking the aid station volunteer about the bathroom over there so I could go hurry her out of it.... the volunteer tells me, "That is not a bathroom, the trail goes up there past the building..." OH shit! Christian and I tear up into the woods like nutcases to catch Kim, not that she really needed us, but just the adrenaline of losing my runner and I was flying like madman uphill. I caught her at the top about halfway through the loop, and we finished it off going back in. We had to be back in to the Grist Mill by 3:47 am because this was a very short loop, but because it is all up and down, and Kim's quads are very sore at this point, she could only climb and descend so fast, and we made it in around 3:50 am.

Kim's 2007 Mohican finished at 75.0 miles counted, and 75.9 miles covered because they don't count the loop you don't make in time. That is around 15 miles farther than she went last year, 7 miles farther than one very seasoned and fit runner I know made it. I cannot help but think if I would have spoken up at the CB to the doctors, we would have been able to start the orange loop at least and maybe get her 80 miles. I know Kim doesn't hold it against me, because she could have spoken up too, and there are many others aspects of her own race that she will discuss on her blog (www.ultranewby.blogspot.com)

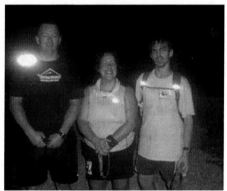

FitfromFat, Kimba, and Christian at the Grist Mill.

Does my race experience end here at the Grist Mill?

Come on, this is me. I came here to run ALL night, and I wanted "Mo" running. So I told Christian I was going out on the **Orange Loop** anyhow because I thought I could pass some runners and maybe pace them further into the race. He wanted to come along. Kim looked at me, knew I was crazy enough to do it, and she and the volunteer there gave me a little shortcut trail to take to help me pass some racers and beat them to the CB so I could see if they wanted pacers. We filled our bottles and took off.

We went into Mohican Campground A and entered Hemlock Grove trail at the back of the campground, after stopping at the ranger station and grabbing a map, and bypassing a hilly section the runners of the race have to do. We ran up the Mohican River to CB and when we got there, the only runners coming in didn't need or want pacers. DAMN. Well, we thought about what to do for a bit, it is now 5am and starting to barely lighten up...a crewmember comes out of the woods and is loading up his truck.... I ask him if he would mind driving us to Rock Point so we could get in front of more runners (hopefully Josh!) and try to get more work pacing. He drives us, me upfront for directions, and Christian sitting in the bed of this S10 pickup.

When we get there I check in with the timer, and I may have misunderstood her, but I THOUGHT she said Josh was already through there. So we ask the next runner if he needs a pacer.... Nope.... then the next..."Hell yeah!!" We got our job. Sean McCormack of Cincinnati (funny that is where Josh is from.) Out we go, and right from the start I can tell we have a smart runner. 90+ miles into this race and he still has the energy to run ALL the down hills and flats and we are only walking the up hills. Many around us are walking everything.... they will still finish but they are wiped out, and Sean is still running.

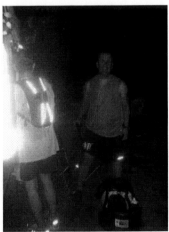

Picking up some part time work with Sean at about 5:45 am.

Sean was a real joy to run with and told us about his 8-day-old first daughter back at home. Quinn Hailey was her name. We just talked

111

and talked and hopefully distracted him a good amount through those final hard miles. Before we knew it we were at Landoll's Castle aid station where I filled his water bottle, and grabbed half of an egg and cheese sandwich...out we go, 5 miles to the finish. I pushed Sean a little bit to challenge himself, but he didn't need it.

Up and down a few more hills...we see Gabe Rainwater from near where Kim lives and I am so shocked because I thought he had dropped.... it must have been another Gabe.

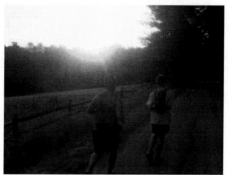

Country Roads, please take me home.

I have Kim's directions in my pocket and have been pulling them out and giving Sean distances to each turn.... we are now on some rural roads to the finish so I have distances to each intersection. At about two miles to go I just put them away and tell Sean "I would keep giving you distances, but it doesn't matter, because you are just going to run it whatever it is!" That got a laugh. The last real climb and descent is Big Hill Road, aptly named. We walk up it, and it is so steep with loose stones and dirt on the down side, that Sean just walks down. Cool. We can see that we are going to finish around 8:30 or so, about a 27:30 for his race. Sean was very appreciative for our company, and Christian and I both felt more grateful to be there witnessing a 100 mile finish with him.

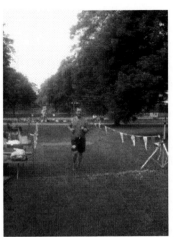
I ran ahead at the end and got pictures for Sean.

After Sean gets in, my wife asks me if I saw Josh out there. What? He is still on the course I am told.

OK, what do you think I would do? I wolfed down a sandwich, and got a ride to find him. I found him cresting Big Hill Rd., and I jumped out and started running with him. We run down Big Hill Rd together, he preferred to run it, and do our best to run as much as possible of Wally Rd to the finish. I got to run maybe a mile and a half with him, and again I darted ahead to get pictures. Even though I was through an hour earlier as a pacer people still freaked out when I took what looked like a wrong turn so I could get in position for photos. I had to shout out "I am a pacer! NOT a racer!" They were trying to help and thought I was running the race.

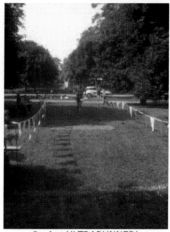
Josh - ULTRARUNNER!

I am so grateful for all the experience I gained this weekend that will go into making me successful in my journeys. From Kim's example, to Vince, Sean, Josh, **Roy**, **Wild Bill Wagner**, and more I will take something with me that will make me better.

Now, I think I am ready to do some Mo Running! Next year I will experience this race as an entrant.

Mohican 100 Trail Race: www.mohican100.org

July would bring many good adventures that are hard to leave out...

SUNDAY, JULY 15, 2007

All Night Running
(and product updates)

As previously reported, my neighbor (and coach) Tony and I planned an all night run to gain nighttime trail running experience in preparation for the BR100. Our plan was to run 9pm until 9am the following morning. We were both mega excited for the adventure...discussing, modifying plans all this past week to make sure we did all we could to be ready. The only hitch in our schedule would be if I got home on a later airline from work and we had to start a little late. As it turns out, I was home by 5:30pm with plenty of time to spare. In fact, too much...I went out to **Red Lobster** for dinner with the family and thinking about how many calories I was going to burn, I decided to eat a lot...and I had stuffed mushrooms, coleslaw, applesauce, 4 of their little biscuits, and a plate with two grilled salmon filets and rice. Plus 3 diet cokes...I know this is HUGE, but honestly that is what I had.... thinking I would need all that energy.

When I got back, I packed way more gear than I needed and WAY more food as I was determined to not run low on fuel again as I have in past long runs. I had 4 pairs of shoes with me to try in case anything bothered me...I had three changes of shirt. Rain was forecast and I wanted to have a few dry shirts in case it soaked us. I packed bodyglide, vaseline, extra underwear, three pair of socks, clif bars, shot blocks, sport beans, and extra (cheapie) headlamp, bug spray, a cooler of sandwiches and fruit, my camera, and three water bottles. Also the S! Caps and Hammer Anti-Fatigue Caps I just bought. More on them later.

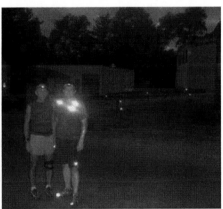

On your mark, get set....photo taken from on top of Vince's Honda Element, thanks Vince!

We started at 9:13 pm after running a hair late.... as we left the parking lot to do our first loop of Pine Lane, we passed two bikers and I remarked that we must keep track of how many people we saw on the trails all night. I knew that most Northeastern Ohio trail runners had blown their wads earlier that day on the Buckeye Trail 50k and I didn't expect to see many, if any at all. We would not see another soul ALL night long until the sun had come up and we were within our last mile of running. We did see our share of wildlife throughout the night. We saw maybe 5-6 deer, a cat in the canal on a log, a few bats buzzing by our heads (our headlamps attracted the bugs they like to eat) and Tony came upon a new friend of ours, that I have never seen in Ohio before.... maybe they are nocturnal.

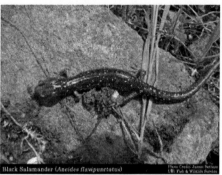

Black Salamander (Aneides flavipunctatus)   Photo Credit: James DeMent
                                                             US Fish & Wildlife Service

Meet my friend, and yours, Mr. Sal A. Mander.

The first loop should have been a breeze, but with all that food sitting in my belly, I was not comfortable.... actually, Tony had the same dilemma, although I think to a lesser extent. Within about a mile and a half, I stopped and fertilized an area just off the trail while Tony walked ahead. We agreed that anytime one of us had to drop a bomb, the other would walk until the pooper could catch up. Mine was the only wilderness poop; we had bathrooms at Boston Store and Pine Lane.

Tony really had a strong desire to get 50 miles in during our planned 12 hours, and I have no doubt I can do that sometime, but NOT tonight. I had issues with not feeling well all night. At times I was sleepy due to a weird and hard work at week flying...other times I felt fatigued and my lower back would ache. I would have to switch between the walking and jogging to get reprieve. The later the night went, the more it felt good to jog instead of walk, which was nice. My feet got real tired of my shoes as well at times. I started in my original pair of green Cascadian.... after 21 miles I switched to an old pair of **Nike Air Alfords**.... after 26 miles I switched into my **North Face** trail shoes.... basically I could tell that I was not capable of the distance Tony wanted on this terrain, feeling like this, at night...my limitations would eventually set the distance we achieved.

A word on nighttime trail running; It is hard to adequately express how much more energy it takes out of you to have to run by headlamp, and look so hard for roots and rocks to avoid tripping on. It REALLY wears you out! Tony actually fell twice tonight, both times while running behind me. His **Gatorade** bottle went flying both times, but always within sight. I really feel for people when they fall. This may be hard to believe but I have only fallen twice that I can remember, while running the Winter BT 50k on a downhill muddy spot that had been trampled into a mushy mess... I also fell on an icy patch during a Saturday morning Southeast Running club training run. I have been very lucky. Must be the Irish in me.

As the night wore on, I became less and less enchanted with finishing this thing out. As far as the anti-fatigue caps go, I had an impression that they were going to make distances I could already do more comfortable. I took the recommended dosage (2-4 one hour prior to exercise and one per hour.) I WAS taking them in combination with my S! Caps (electrolytes) and I don't know if there is any conflict there. Basically what I noticed was that my hardest hours were after I had taken the Anti-Fatigue caps, and on the hours when I skipped them to experiment, I was a little more upbeat and running more. This is not the death knoll for them in my opinion; I will try them on another run without S! Caps while using something else for electrolytes like **Gatorade**. I will not mess with them anymore prior to BR100 though, and definitely NOT in the race.

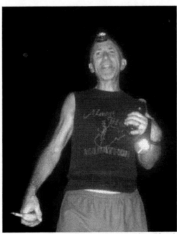

Tony the Tiger during one of our early stops...there's the flying **Gatorade**!

Many times during my hardest periods, I wanted to tell Tony that when we got back to the car, I was going to sleep while he ran a loop alone and see if that helped. Generally, I kept my mouth shut and by the time we got back to the car I was feeling better and kept moving. During our last loop it was getting harder. I laid down on the cellar door by the ranger station for about 5 minutes to try to relieve my back, and then I ate a sandwich, changed shoes again (to the **North Face**) and I actually felt pretty jazzy for the first mile to mile and a half before slippng back into struggling again. The thing that got me up and moving for our third Pine Lane Loop (taking us to 34 miles) was the thought that I wasn't going to let the whole "death before dawn" syndrome stop me. This is where they say for 100 milers the hardest time to get through is the last two hours before dawn. (It is always darkest just before the dawn, right?)

I thought about the prospect of stopping at 4:30 am, and how I would feel race day and I said to myself, "Hell no!" I will not be taken down tonight, or on race day in that fashion. I know in my brain that this dilemma exists, so I can overcome it. You know what? I did that last loop...halfway through, at Pine Lane trailhead, I had to sit down for about 5 minutes on a bench there....just recouping and getting remotivated...well, the sun was coming up now, about 6 am or so and when I headed back down the trail that first mile or two again really had me motivated. I wanted to get back to the car and crank out another Pine Lane loop to take us to 42 miles in 12 hours or so. I relented though, and as I got closer I realized that I KNOW I can do the distance, and I will have days where I can do it MUCH easier than this night....I wanted to call it a day/night/day at 34 miles and start recovering the body. I think I will get more from stopping early last night and recovering than from doing that extra 8 miles. It was in me, but for what advantage?

I had another problem on the last loop that I have heard about and not experienced much thankfully. Early on in that last 8 mile loop I realized I was getting a case of **Baboon Butt** and wouldn't have any relief until I got back to the end of the loop. I just had to bear it.

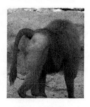

We finished at 07:11 just about 10 hours after we started.... we ran through the entire **night** (seeing no one!) and we beat the death before dawn! Our pace was just what it would take to finish in 30 hours, but we also ran some of the hardest terrain we will see in the race all night, and our aid stations were not manned.... and it was **all** at night...I regret that we did not go the whole 12 hours one on level, and am proud I had the courage to stop as well. It may mean something positive for my BR100 race that I didn't punish myself too bad this evening. Immediately after finishing I mixed and drank a bottle of Recoverite, which Hammer sent as a sample with my caps. I do think that this probably does something to help me recover quicker and more fully.

Tony was upbeat about what we did accomplish, and it was fun watching everyone show up at Boston Store for their morning run, and we were covered in dirt and sweat and had been running since they all went to bed the night before! We met a runner who said he was about to register for BR100, which is the second time I have met someone at Boston Store claiming that lately. Josh and I ran into a guy that said the same thing. The guy this night was named Pat McDaniels (I think I got it right) and has done three Mohican 100's (best time 22 hours and change) and said his training for previous 100 milers was all 10-12 mile runs because of time constraints. I was amazed by this, but he talked about how he would run them harder to get more out of them, and I will have to think about it...In any case, I will be watching the entrant list for him to sign up! He seemed very nice.

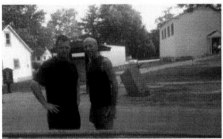

Finish Line Photos! Tony, if you want a 5x7 framed copy, I will be glad to charge you 55 dollars like the photos from the marathons! Call me.

At some point in the night, it came upon me that I had finally found a color for Tony for my blog. He is Tony the Tiger, and he is GREEEAAATTT! He was so upbeat and supportive and loyal to me during the run. Tony values his running friendships so highly I almost can't put it into words. I heard so many stories all night about different running relationships he has had over the years and adventures they have had. Knowing how much he talks about me, and how valuable he makes me feel as a friend it just a true treasure. Today, I went into Second Sole wanting to try on a GPS watch I am salivating over (Suunto x9i) and I ran into Leo who works there and who Tony had talked about just last night, and Leo tells me how much Tony talks about his neighbor!!! OK, confessional here (Vince, you will have to understand...) I bought a pair of shoes at Second Sole because Vertical Runner doesn't carry the Pearl Izumi brand. I have wanted to try them for some time, since talking to Roger about how much he likes his. I had a coupon emailed to me from Active.com for Fleet Feet to get 20% off and I tried some on in Second Sole, because I wanted to know if it was worth driving up there for the shoes.... well Leo said they will honor the coupon there, so what the heck? The shoe whore strikes once more!!!

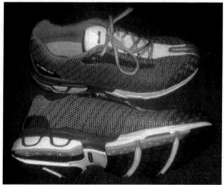

Pearl Izumi **Synchrofloat**....perhaps for the **Akron marathon**?

OK, one more product announcement from the FitfromFat photography department. I invested about 23 dollars in a tripod with flexible legs to allow me all kinds of choices while shooting photos on the run! I can fold the legs together and the whole deal will fit in my pocket.

I am very excited about my next planned run, I am supposed to run 2 hours or so with Roy Heger on Tuesday. I am going to try to more or less interview him, and pick his brain for pace help for BR100!

Roy Heger

So, it came to my devious little brain that I needed more time in the company of an ultra veteran who has a lot of wisdom to share. After witnessing his 10th finish at the **Mohican 100** June 17, earning him his 1000 mile buckle. I kind of wanted to interview Roy as much as run with him. I intend on running with many ultra veterans if they will run with me and kind of making that a series on the blog. My next target is Connie Gardner, who I don't really know at all, but *everyone* knows is a fantastic runner from Ohio. You don't talk about women runners in the area without hearing her name. She was first female at **Mohican**, first female at the Buckeye Trail 50k Saturday, and on and on...She is currently getting ready to run a large 24 hour race...maybe I can talk to her before that.... Roy knows her, and I am going to ask his help to arrange it.

It rained the whole time I was driving there, but since I was going West from where I lived it worked out that by the time I got there I had passed under all the rain and it stayed more or less dry for the run. There were some moments that sounded like rain from the canopy above in the woods, but I think it was mostly previous rainfall amongst the leaves, as we never really got wet.

Well I arrived at the Hinckley Reservation at the agreed upon hour of 6pm to find Roy prepping himself, and his wife Theresa prepping JD their Thoroughbred/Arab gelding for his trail run. Roy and I would go our way while JD and Theresa went theirs, with us meeting back up with around 2.5 miles to go at the end. I think Theresa had the better-looking running partner; JD was a very nice looking horse. Sorry Roy! **Don't be so long in the face**, I am just teasing you!

We motored out and I quickly got in a few pacing questions off my planned script, but as could be expected, we also rambled off topic quick as you can imagine. It can be hard to direct the conversation where you want it to go without being rude. I am not the kind of person to be like that (I hope) and as Roy was giving me history lessons on the landmarks of this particular area I tried to soak it in, returning to my questions as long pauses would permit. I can at least report that as I related my plans for running the BR100, Roy never stopped mid trail, turned around and asked "Are you nuts!?!?!" So, that could be a good sign. He confirmed an idea I have had in my mind for some time about this race. I am **not** going to wear a watch. I am going to run what I can run, walk what I need to walk, and just have a nice day! In and out of the aid stations with minimal time down...eat on the walk/run while moving out. Bottles filled ahead of time and exchanged for empties at every aid station where crew is permitted.

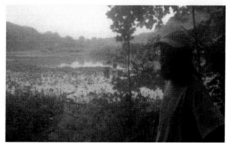

By the man made lake in Hinckley...there is a **great blue heron** behind Roy.

We ran by an area called the boathouse where you can rent rowboats, paddleboats, and canoes. I will going back there with the girls soon! At some point shortly after this last photo, we ran into one of Roy's high school peers and stopped for a brief chat. As it turns out her name is Marina (sp?) and that made me giggle that I met Marina by the lake.

We found some decidedly tough hills on the way up to Whipp's Ledges and just ran up them. I only walked once, when it was so steep that walking was as fast or faster. I ran an amazing amount of uphill tonight, and loved it!

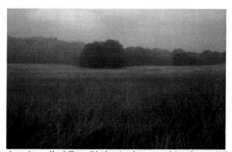

This little meadow is called Top O' the Ledges and is above Whipp's Ledges.

Whipp's Ledges is an area with cliffs and ledges (formed of Sharon conglomerate) similar to the Gorge I run in and the Ledges area by Kendall Lake. There are two other ledges areas in Hinckley which I did not see, and will have to go back to check out. According to Roy, one of them has some very neat relief carvings.

122

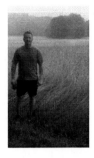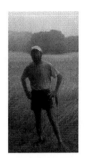

No flat areas to set a camera up near here, and I forgot my Gorillapod thingie tonight....so individual pictures have to do.

We ran on for awhile talking about all kinds of folks Roy has run with: Connie Gardner, Kim Martin, Mark and Stephen Godale, Wild Bill Wagner, and on and on. Roy told me the story about one year when the local cross country team made it to State and he had promised if they made it to State he would run to the meet in Columbus, and he did. His comments about running on the road reminded me of how much I detest running on the roadside and made me wonder why I have been daydreaming about running coast to coast.....

I learned a few new things from Roy not related to running. The photo below is of a building on a farm we ran by and he casually referred to it as a summer kitchen. I latched onto that and asked him about the terminology and he said that is what these little side buildings commonly are on farms.

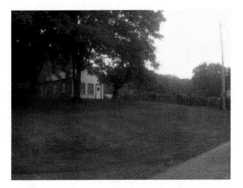

Then right after this, we backtracked a few hundred feet up the road to see this **GIANT anchor** and capstan (below.) The capstan is the

123

little blue and white knob in the foreground. Sailors would put large poles into the holes in it and wind the **anchor** up and down via the windlass (not shown.) I was just focused on not messing up the peoples flowers while Roy shot the photo...

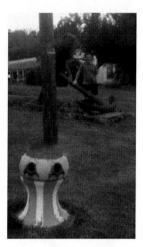

We moved on down the road from here talking about our mutual love for aviation (I would love to take Roy flying.) This then morphed into a discussion about our love for hot rods. Which ended up with me telling Roy about the Cobra my Dad and I built, and hopefully I can take him out for a ride some time.

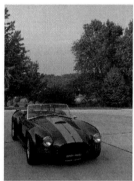

My Dad and I handbuilt this car from a kit. It is a hoot and I am always looking for an excuse to drive it. The style is called a **Shelby Cobra**, but it is a replica and not an original.

A little while later we ran into Theresa and JD when we turned back onto the bridle trail and would run back to the cars with them. I learned a lot about running with horses and not spooking them, and why they spook. Roy tells me that when it comes to "fight or flight" horses are pretty much stuck with "flight" because they have little to defend themselves with. So, like deer, horses are very sensitive to threats and very quick to get out of there if they feel threatened. JD was a little like this and Theresa was saying that tonight he was afraid of his own shadow. He did fine around me though and I made sure he could see me as I passed him at any time. We passed a large rock on the side of the road that they told me one night it took him 10 tries to pass because it scared him.

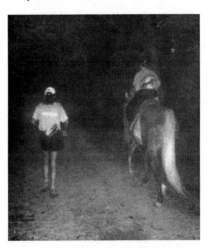

Whose "tail" is longer? Roy's ponytail or JD's horsetail? Well at least Roy's "tail" isn't white...I had the impression for some reason that Roy was 59 and when he talked about his upcoming 54th birthday I challenged him saying he was attempting to "bullshit a bullshitter." Well he wasn't, I must have been thinking of Fred Davis who is 59 (and a future interview prospect along with his supportive and funny wife!)

To my surprise we were able to run faster than JD, especially because he is younger and can't run the down hills yet. We waited up for them several times, once when we crossed a stream and he had to drink (he should go to Vince for a Nathan bottle, or even a hydration pack!) The last mile had a good amount of uphill where JD is stronger than us, and we were pushing ourselves to keep up with him. I don't know how it got started, but we just seemed to keep running harder and harder. Near the top I proclaimed that I had an extra gear to Roy and burst ahead to catch up to JD, just to see if I actually did. I didn't pass him as I both didn't want to spook him on this spot, and didn't know the way we were going....I was shocked at what I had left in my legs after all this climbing. We were judiciously rewarded with a long downhill to the car where both Roy and I let our legs stretch and carry us at a fairly prodigious pace. Somewhere about halfway down he says this is what Kim Martin or Connie Gardner would run like for the whole run.....oh man! I hope I can catch Connie on a slow run, or just take her out to lunch and interview her! That speed for two hours would kill me!!!

My thanks to Roy and Theresa for accomodating me, teaching me about horses and the Hinckley area, and having fun! Roy made an offhand comment that maybe he would help me (pace me?) through my first Mohican 100 next year as he is done running Mohican for a little while now that he has done 10. He has 8 Massanutten 100s and will whip that goal next of running 10 there. He has already helped me immensely, whether he will admit it or not, and he just set a new goal of mine in **stone**. I will run the 2009 Massanutten (Roy's 10th) as my first. I hope it shows through in my post that I have immense respect for Roy because I *do*.

TUESDAY, JULY 24, 2007

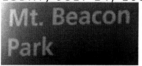

My workday got cut a little short today and I ended up back in Newburgh, NY. Normally we stay right in Newburgh at the Hampton Inn but tonight they got us a rental car and we went across the river in Fishkill, NY just south of Poughkeepsie. Since we had a rental car, AND I was done earlier in the day, I thought I would try to find a trail to run on in some of the hills around here. The desk staff at the hotel advised me of a trail in the Hudson Highlands State Park which goes up Mt. Beacon. A quick change out of the monkey suit and into my gear and I was off like a prom dress!

It was only about a 20 minute drive to the trailhead and fortuitously there is a convenience store right there. Bob's Country Corner or something like that. I purchased a Grape Gatorade to fulfill my sponsorship obligations and a pack of Fig Newtons to fulfill my addiction. They weren't the whole grain ones though, so it was kind of ok, not transcendental....

The first part of the trail seemed nice and runnable and I was going to try to run up this behemoth at a very slow pace.... then came the steps. Looming out of the woods was a set of steps, there must have been 100 or more. They were built on a steel frame and the steps themselves were almost all concrete slabs spanning the frame. It was kind of weird looking. Occasionally a step was replaced by a wooden one, telling me that sometimes the concrete ones must get brittle and crack. I started walking about halfway up these.

At the top of the steps was Massanutten. Or Hardrock. Or Mountain Masochist. This trail was so DAMN rocky that it made me think immediately that it must be what these mountain races are like. It was quite steep too, so with the combination I was running very little of the uphill now. Just trying not to twist an ankle and keep walking at a good forward pace like I must do in the BR100. There are NO sections like this in the BR though, thankfully.

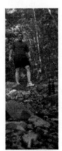
Mountain Mike

The trail would switch back and forth, very common for trails going up mountain sides. There were the occasional offshoots and this trail was not marked in any fashion that I was aware of, so at every junction I was making a mental note of some landmark, so I could find my way back to the car. I didn't have any fixed time or distance goal in mind, but I knew I wanted to make it to the top of this trail, and if that didn't take too long, linger around up there looking for flat trails to run before coming back down.

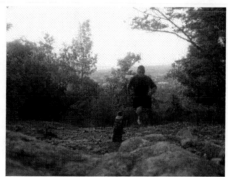

I WAS thinking on the way up that this is good training for some of the harder mountain races.

As you can tell, I took some pictures on the way up. I call these ultra pictures because I take the pictures when I am going up and walking, and then run all the downhill, taking no pictures. If you run ultras you know what I mean.

The first level at the top was a real treat...it was kind of an intermediate level off with ledges and an old abandoned industrial type building that kids obviously party in. The view from here over the Hudson Valley was beautiful. A few hours later and deeper into the sunset it must have been truly remarkable.

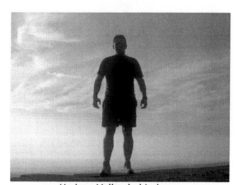

Hudson Valley behind me.

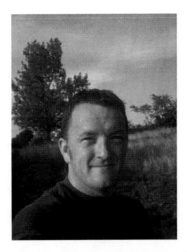

At this intermediate type summit, I could tell that there was still some of the mountain left to climb. I headed of down a much more level, runnable trail and explored several different side loops a short way, before finding the one path that led up, up, up all the way.

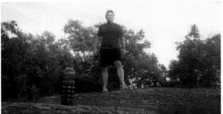

Notice it is not just **Gatorade**...it is **FIERCE Gatorade**! I love it. It is the same damn stuff in the bottle as regular **Gatorade**.

I ran into the antenna farm that currently serves the area for several radio stations and apparently TV stations. I ran into an abandoned antenna site where I was able to get inside the building and see all the equipment left behind.... and then the trail wound up all the way to the summit. Beyond yet another abandoned antenna station I was shocked as I wound my way past the building to see an obelisk. Now THAT demands some extra investigation.

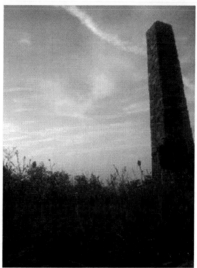

The Obelisk at the Summit of Mt. Beacon

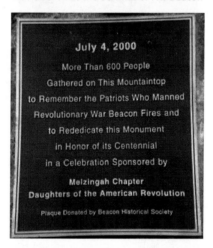

July 4, 2000

More Than 600 People
Gathered on This Mountaintop
to Remember the Patriots Who Manned
Revolutionary War Beacon Fires and
to Rededicate this Monument
in Honor of its Centennial
in a Celebration Sponsored by

Melzingah Chapter
Daughters of the American Revolution

Plaque Donated by Beacon Historical Society

As I got closer I noticed a plaque attached to the obelisk...OK, looks like there was a ceremony up here July 4th, 2000 to rededicate the obelisk...nice, but it didn't tell my WHY there was an obelisk....

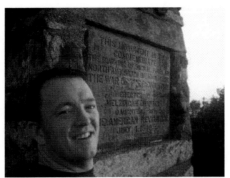

Notice the date of **July 4th**, 1900, 100 years before the plaque on the other side.

Then I went around to the side facing the valley, and saw this original carving that opened my eyes. The mountain is called beacon, because they used it as such to warn of invading troops I guess. Hence Mt. Beacon, and also the name of the town my car was parked in was Beacon. Cool huh? I was wondering for awhile how many locals know why their town is called Beacon and whether any school teachers bring their classes up here to show them this. I would if I was a teacher!

On the way back down the hill, I was able to run much more of the trail walking only when the rocks got so *ubiquitous* that I feared turning an ankle or sliding downhill. What took me an hour and 20 minutes going uphill and farting around taking all the pictures, took me 25 minutes going downhill, and taking just two photos. It really does open my eyes to what some of the harder mountain races are going to be like to try running on a small mountain like this!

Wildlife Report: On the way up the mountain I did encounter one young deer, and in keeping with Josh's deer project goals, I started to go off trail to see how close I could get. I took ONE step of the side of the trail, dislodged a rock, and the fawn was gone. I got to maybe 100 feet from it...

On the way back down the mountain, I saw what I thought was a mole skittering across the trail and then he got kind of caught up trying to get over some rocks and I got a good look at him, but couldn't get the camera out in time. After looking at photos of moles on Google, I am not so sure, so I will not put a photo up. It was like a long dark mouse basically, but didn't have the claws and pale nose of a mole. Too bad, he was going to be named Vinny the Mole. I might have even made him a honorary cousin of mine.

Clarence Fahnestock State Park

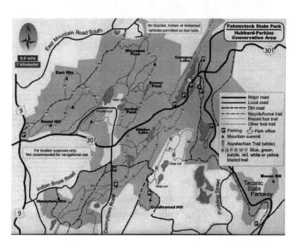

The plan is to get up about 30 minutes before sunrise and drive to the Clarence Fahnestock State Park for a run of approximately 2 hours. I duty on at 11 am so if I am running by 6 am or so and done by 8 am, then I can be back by 8:30 in time to shower, eat and be ready for the airport. I am writing this first paragraph the night before and have to say that the part that has me excited the most is seeing some of the Appalachian Trail (AT.) So many adventures have occurred on this 2174-mile trail, which connects Springer Mountain, Georgia to Baxter Peak in Katahdin, Maine. The maps are printed, the camera battery is charging and I am about to go to bed!

Wake up: I didn't REALLY want to get out of bed at 5 something am...I had stayed up a little later messing around down by the hotel desk, getting the above map printed so I would know where I was in the park. First the hotel business center printer would not work.... then we rebooted everything and it still didn't work.... but by now the desk clerk had heard some of my story and why I wanted a map, and he let me come behind the desk and print my map from there. Got to bed around 1 am or so....after laying everything out, INCLUDING toilet paper pre-folded and in the pockets of my shorts I couldn't forget.

I DID get up though, and like always, I am now *so* glad I did. I didn't make the actual sunrise, but today it was a little overcast, so I don't

132

think I missed all that much. I had a handful of cashews and headed out for Fahnestock (pronounced like "Waynestock".... schwinnng!) About a 15-minute drive as expected and when I got there, I was not at first sure I had the right parking area. Then I found the first marker on the trail and I knew I was there.

The plan was to park at the second parking area down Dennytown Rd. and start by running out to the Northeast on the AT, and then return along the Blue trail (marked in a square with a B on the map) to the car. I wasn't sure how far I could get with the time available this morning and the fact that I only wanted to run two hours in taper, but I figured I would find out. Of course I imagined I could make it all the way to the large lake along 301, but as is usually the case with trails, it was slower going than I imagined. First time on the trail, and stopping for photos, tends to make progress occur a little more slowly.

Entering the Appalachian Trail for my first time, I couldn't help but to spend some time thinking about those who had tread this soil before me, most notably David Horton. He held the record for the fastest transit of the AT for quite some time, and I just watched his movie about setting the record on the Pacific Crest Trail (PCT) called "The Runner." I was wondering what time of day he came through where I was, what the weather was, and how many days he still had ahead of him til he got to the finish. I honestly don't know whether he did his trek going Northbound or Southbound.

Anyways, back to my trek. This trail was much rockier than anything we run in Ohio, but at the same time slightly less rocky than the Mt. Beacon trail of the other night. I was able to run most of the trail here if I was careful...maybe 80%. There were still sometimes where the rocks were so plentiful and closely spaced, that the best option was just to slow to a walk and pick my way through.

The wildlife didn't waste much time in presenting itself to me today. The first thing I saw out of the car was three wild roosters. They were just wandering around the field by the trailhead. Once I got into the woods and started to sweat a little bit, it took me no time to lament the absence of any bug spray on my body. My arms may have gotten as strenuous a workout as my legs today, with the swatting of all those damn flies. I won't linger on the topic of the flies (horseflies?) but let me just say this....To all my friends running or pacing at the BR100, who might be worried about flies and bugs, don't worry. They are apparently **ALL** in the Hudson Valley of New York State. :-)

Around 20 minutes down the trail, some little hoppy guy jumps across the bow of my Nikes and I stopped to investigate. As I made my friends with this little guy, the first name that came to my mind was Montgomery.

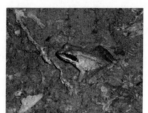

Montgomery the Fahnestock Frog.

Now, keeping with the hoppy theme, I am about 15 minutes further down the AT and walking up a fairly steep and rocky uphill and I see Archibald's cousin from the East Coast. If you will recall, Archibald is from Minneapolis (a similar toad I found on a river in Minneapolis in another post.) His cousin Albert was here to see me today, and graciously posed for a photo.

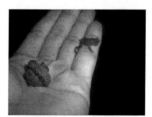

Albert the tiny toad.

The really funny thing to me after I took this photo is this: I put that acorn in my hand thinking it would give some scale to the tiny size of Albert. Then I was laughing at myself thinking that anyone can see my fingers and gauge the scale from there...the thought that came to me is that some readers may think that I have Hagrid hands and that the toad is actually full size. (Give me a break; the Hagrid reference is chronologically appropriate right now, OK?)

Now, I had no IDEA when I got up this morning that I was going to see my friend Tony on the run. Had I known, I would have been SOOOO excited. But there I was, about 15 minutes after Albert and about to make a turn on the trail, and I look ahead and there is Tony, scampering across the trail...Well, I immediately said hi and started to engage him in conversation, etc. We both stopped what we were doing to hang out a while, although eventually we had to part ways again. I really wanted to take **Tony** back to Ohio and I was SURE he would have liked going, but it just wasn't practical today for us.

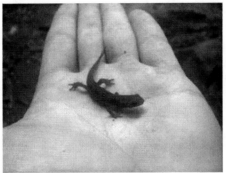

Tony, *__my favorite trail find of all time__*, wildlife speaking.

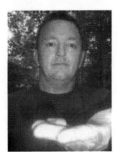

Me and **Tony**!!!

Finding this little guy, and holding him really mesmerized me. He was very accommodating and didn't seem to mind too much when I picked him up and moved him around. I will have to look him up on Wikipedia and see if he is a salamander or newt or what. I actually have a plan to get two of these guys tattooed on my right arm, on top of an autumn leaf fairly soon. I probably spent between 5-10 minutes playing with **Tony** before **gingerly** putting him down off the side of the trail.

When I popped out at the first intersection between the AT and the **Blue trail**, I had to go ahead and head back towards the car...I didn't have a whole lot of extra time to play with, and needed to get back in time to be available in case work needed me. The run back was productive (outside of swatting at flies) and I moved pretty well. On the trail for me, it seems like every run has a mix of those stretches where you lumber along and then those transcendental patches of trail where all the foot falls hit in between rocks or roots naturally and everything is feeling good. I push through the mucky patches to find those idyllic periods when everything is feeling wonderful.

On the way back along the blue trail, I ran into one more picture worthy friend along the trail and he was a funny one. I was hearing this buzzing (which I was growing accustomed to with the DAMN flies) but this was different tone. It would buzz and stop, buzz and stop. I stopped to investigate and then I saw it. A **dragonfly** would fly a short way, hit a tree, fly a short way, hit a tree, etc. Finally, he hit one too hard I guess, and he fell to the forest floor to realign his gyroscopes. There he posed while I got a few shots. I have no idea what was causing him to behave the way he did...maybe he and *Tony* were out drinking a little too late last night, and he was FWI (flying while intoxicated.) My copilot thinks maybe he was just sick.

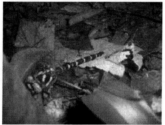

Neville the intrepid flyer. Grounded by the FAA for awhile (Fahnestock Aeronautics Authority)

Trail Markings: This is the cool part. Even though I was in totally unfamiliar territory, I really had no problem following the trail. The markings on this part of the AT were very similar to the Buckeye Trail back home with white blazes the same size as the Buckeye Blue blazes and occasionally little aluminum diamonds nailed to a tree. In addition there were these little round dots attached to trees fairly often which marked the trail. The convention for turns was the same as the Buckeye Trail where they stagger two markings diagonally to indicate the direction of a turn.

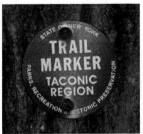

The dot.

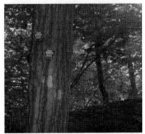

The turn. In this case, a left turn. The upper marking is
Always the way you turn. Blazes on this tree too.

After while, the act of following the blue trail on the way back to the car, became as simple as a game of connect the dots. Similar to the way some of our *races* are marked in Ohio, these trail markers were so frequent that from any one marker you could usually see the next one ahead of it, and the one behind, in case you are going the other way....

I did have one short spot where I had to backtrack and double check that I was still on the blue trail, which I was...the trail just goes through a short poorly marked stretch where it also borders a small lake, and I wasn't sure I hadn't missed a turn. Turns out I hadn't and I then kept going again til the car. There was a lot of trail in this state park that I did not get to see today. I would love to have the regular chance to run these trails from time to time, and I am sure I would be much faster each time through, knowing the way, and not needing to stop every little stretch for pictures. Today wasn't about fast anyways, I am in taper, remember!

Chapter 7 – The 100 Miler, a true ultra test

It is time to take a crack at the 100 miler myself. Am I ready? I know mentally I am. I spend a lot of time in late June and July preparing myself. I sit in the sauna at the gym for increasing amounts of time each day to get my body heat acclimated for the expected HOT conditions of an early August race day.

I *think* I have the race plan all figured out. I know which shoes I am going to wear. I know where my wife will meet me at the aid stations/crew locations to resupply me (and motivate me.) August comes and it is time to experience it for real!!

SATURDAY, AUGUST 04, 2007

Inaugural Burning River 100

- A run through the woods with Harry Potter -

Where do I begin and where do I end? The excitement built and built for my first ever 100-mile race. I really had all the good vibes going into this day, with success on my training runs, happy feelings about my gear selection, a great mental map of the entire course.... I really was mentally in the groove that all the pieces were in place for my first 100 miler. I envisioned running down that last segment of Front street into the Riverwalk square in downtown Cuyahoga Falls with my daughters on either side of me.... beaming.

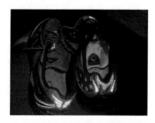

The shoes, the shoes. My original plan was to run the early stages of the race in the shoes on the left (size 12 - 2006 Brooks Cascadia) and then the day before the race I put them on to wear around a little and break them in more, and I noticed that the tongue is not gusseted over to the sides of the shoe like the 2007 model. I know from experience on the course that I can get grit and pebbles down in my shoe, and I wasn't wearing Gaters (ankle wraps that keep grit out) so I chose to go with the 2007 greenies that are gusseted and a size 12.5 to allow for feet expansion, etc. I still put three other pairs of shoes into the trunk of the car in case at one of the crewed aid stations where my wife would be, I wanted to change.

The lights. I would use no light at the start (5am) because the first 9.6 miles is on road....and easy to follow. By the time I hit the woods, around 7am, it would be light. For the night to come, I packed a Petzl headlamp, a Energizer headlamp with the band loosened all the way up which fit around my waist, and a flashlight to be clamped into my water bottle sleeve by my wife when darkness approached with plastic zip ties. This setup, by the way, worked "Brilliant!" (Imagine Ron Weasley's voice here - bear with me, you will see why....)

The clothing. I would wear trusty compression (light squeeze) type underwear under Target C9 running shorts, with a C9 sleeveless mesh type shirt to keep me cool. Once we started this was plenty to keep me warm even at 5am. Socks were Smartwool runnings socks. I also bought a new Halo headband which has a little rubber strip to keep sweat out of the eyes during endurance events....it worked pretty well...

The lube. Yes, the lube. I got up at 2:45 am to leave the house at 3:15 and showered quickly then lubed the feet with bodyglide, the crotch with bodyglide, the nips with bodyglide, the armpits with BG, and yes, the buttcrack of dawn with BG. I also carried Vaseline in the crew bag in case I felt like changing or just doing between my toes.

The calories. Besides what I would find at the very well stocked aid stations, I brought along one pack of Clif Shot blocks for the first 10 miles as well as two gels (which I hate eating, but they work.) In the crewbag were about 7 Odwalla energy bars of various flavors. Before leaving the house, I downed a Muscle Milk with protein and a banana...I think that was it.

The friends. This should really be the first category as it is the most important by far (but then I couldn't insert this sentence to make that point, could I?) Josh had showed up (ON TIME! OMFG!!!) at noon on Friday at my house. I bought lemonade from my daughter's lemonade stand. So did Tony by the way...Kim! She arrives! I am always SO excited to catch up with these people. It feels like Christmas every time I see them.

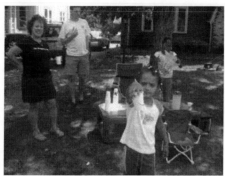

Want some Lemonade? They could have run an aid station! They made **27 dollars** selling lemonade.

We would meet up with Josh's pacer Adam at the pre-race briefing, as well as Tony Mathison from Baines, TX who would be sharing the ultra-luxurious surface of my living room floor as race accomodations. Adam is an ultrarunner himself and works for a running store down in Cincy....Tony has done a few 100's, I think if I remember right, Rocky Racoon (my next planned) as well as Lean Horse, and some 100+ mile runs at ATY (a fixed time race in the Phoenix area every year at New Year's - just watch Josh's blog, he is trying to get in....)

Josh should be well known to regular reader's of this blog, but if not, go back and catch up, or over to his blog. He is the hottie with a naughty body that all the Northeastern Ohio lady runners get caught salivating over. You know who you are ladies!

Tony, my ultra-marathon neighbor, was there. Christian, who paced Kim with me at Mohican, would be at the race. Sean McCormack who we also paced at Mo would be there. Rob Powell, Bill Wagner, Roy Heger, Chef Bill Bailey, Tanya Cady, Regis Shivers Jr., Lloyd, Vince, Mel, Fred Davis (first time 100 miler! - inside media joke....), Joe the race director, Mike Helkovich, Leo Lightner and probably some I can't remember now (sorry..) I found that I was excited to just get to that pre-race meeting and dinner and meet everyone again! Really.

I already know what the running part is like. We show up, put on our shoes, and see how long we can do it. And that is what the weekend was about, but for some reason I was just jazzed to see everyone again.

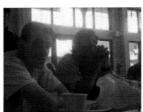

Josh D! and Tony from TX. Tony may have been the most perfectly polite runner of the whole weekend! I cannot tell you what a kind and gentle man he is in mere words!

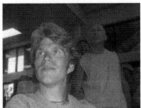

Adam from Cincinnati (Kim, do the eyes approach the league of Alabama Andy?) **Tony the Tiger**, ready to break the chains and roar to his first 100-mile finish, he did **GGGREEEAAATTTT!**

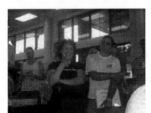

Tom Jennings (my heat guru - and hopefully a future training partner....Tom?) and the Goddess! Kim!

The pre-race dinner (from Bill Bailey) was excellent. Whole grain pasta with marinara and meatballs, salads, cookies, bread.... assorted drinks. I was pretty aware of everything that was coming down the pike as far as race announcements so it was mostly social hour until it was over, and then back to the house with Josh, Adam, and Tony to try to get some sleep before the race. I get in the car with Kim to go back and my phone, which I had silenced, has several messages. First my Dad, "Mike, it's your Dad, call me when you get this." Then, my sister "Mike, it's Anne. Mom is in the hospital with a problem with one of her lungs, call me if you want when you get this...." What? I know she hasn't been feeling well, but didn't expect this.

141

I call my Dad, and he is much more calm than myself after hearing this. He says it wasn't ambulatory and they sent her over for further tests after an x-ray at a doctor's appointment showed a portion of one lung collapsed. I asked him, well, is this an emergency type visit or just checking? Is there anything I can do? I am wondering if starting this race is the right thing to do now or what? He says, "Mike, run the race. You can't do anything right now, it is not an emergency, and she is ok, just in for tests for now. She wants you to run your race." OK, but damn, this is my MOM man.... she has smoked since before me.... and there is an issue in a lung? That doesn't feel good. Not at all.

All I could do was to rely on my wife to keep me updated at the crewing locations, and if something were worse than expected, I would just pull out of the race and head South to the hospital. She was going to be in tests all day, and I honestly thought the only therapy that would really soothe my worry would be the run anyhow. Running can do that for me.

Go home. A few last minute prep items.... and I am to bed before 10pm. Somehow the whole pre race jitters don't come and I am asleep right away. Kind of like when you wear out your kids all day and they just fall right asleep...I think the pre race stresses, coupled with the worries about my Mom, just put me right out.

Awake at 2:45, momentarily wondering why I am up.... then "Oh yeah! Race day..." then "Oh yeah...Mom.... damn." Shower, check on the floor gang, they are all up and nearly ready. I grab my carefully laid out gear.... and away we go! Arrive at the castle at about 4:15, right on time...remembering how important it is to check in so as not to delay race start, I go straight away to Vince and get crossed off the list. Walking back I run into **Tony the Tiger**.... we are both jazzed!

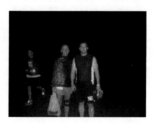

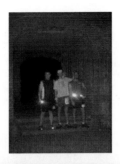

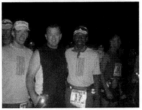

It is so exciting to be about to embark on this journey. We ALL know there is pain ahead. We all are willing to risk the pain for something that matters to each of us. Probably a *different* something for each of us. Shortly before 5am, the National Anthem is sung by someone live, a pretty good job too. Then we are off!

Onto the road, headed south, chatting, etc. Josh is wearing my watch. I wasn't going to wear it anyhow, and he needed one, so he gets it. After less than a mile, one runner is over on the other side stopping to bend over to stretch, or tie a shoe or something, and I shout out "It's early! Don't drop yet! It gets better!" Giggles all around. I run with Texas Tony, leapfrogging him as he does a run/walk strategy. I run with Monica from Illinois. I run leapfrogging Don Clark from MN who has this enormous beard out in front of him. Very ZZ Top, or Mountain Dwarf depending on what your background is.... I really would like to have gotten a picture of him. I am not carrying my camera, just two water bottles, a few snacks in the pockets as well as a Ziploc with S! Caps and a few Advil just in case. I can't remember why, but I have seen warnings not to use too much Advil on ultra races.

I am just in a gentle cruise down Chagrin River Rd. As per my plan, I am turning in about 12 minute miles I think...expecting to get to Polo Fields, 9.6 miles, at about 7:00 am. I have given Lasheda (my wife) a pace chart and maps, and it is marked for a 28 hour pace. That was the plan for the whole day. On a microcosm, however, I kind of forgot that the first segments were going to be much quicker. I skipped the first aid station at 4.7 miles because my bottles were more than half full and I had food in the pockets. I found at 9.6 miles I was ready for a good poop, and stood in line for 3-4 minutes for the john. I had arrived there in 1:51 so there was no hurry. But it is a race, and even at a 100 miler, I couldn't help but feel hurried. I think I will grow out of that.

I got to run and talk with Rob a lot in the first 10 miles, but my bathroom break insures he is long gone when I am back out with full water bottles, a few snacks and on my way. I did get to see Don Clark more over the first dirt section from 9.6 to 15.1 and beyond. By the time we are 12-15 miles in, we are getting spaced out and more solitude is available, and I turn to the mp3 player for some company. What shall I listen to? Harry Potter of course! The new book. I had read roughly 300 pages so far, so I moved forward in the audio book to where I had been reading and settled in for the tale.

Out of Harper Ridge (15.1) I am still feeling good, but realizing that I have been going a wee bit fast over the first eighth of the race, so I try to dial back. I didn't do that very well. I should have just walked until I felt like I was back in my pace range. I kept running the runnables and walking the uphills. Shortly before 18.4 miles I see a minivan slow alongside the road, and I look over to see Mack Bell, a guy I went to grade school with, and got surprised by at the Endurance 50 with Dean Karnazes last fall. He had decided to bring his kids out to check out the race and come find me. I got to Shadow Lake (18.4) a full hour ahead of the 28 hour pace. Not by plan, and with no thoughts of a glorious surprising sub24 hour finish, just inexperienced me running a race. Well, Lasheda was here at the first crew access point, and the plan was to have the spare water bottles filled, and I grab them and move on. She was sleeping in the car. Could I blame her? I WAS an hour ahead of when I had written down for her to expect me, and I did make her wakeup at like 3am. I retreat to the aid tables, fill the bottles, holler at Roy, and just as I am leaving the aid station I look back and see Mack and the kids. I was so taken up by doing the necessities at the aid station I forgot to at least stop for a minute and say hi. I hollered back to him that I was sorry we didn't talk more - I really felt bad...but it was also time to keep going forward...

Turn Harry back on and I am down the trail listening to the story. Doing good, but towards the end of this next section I start feeling discomfort in my left hip. Damn, not good, this is the feeling that caused me to drop at the Winter Buckeye Trail 50k last January. Hadn't felt it since. Well it comes and goes, and I have spurts of running. Out of Alexander Rd. aid station it is more prevalent and I take a Walmart type bag filled with ice and just put it against my hip held there by the elastic on the shorts. If it is muscular it should respond to ice I am thinking.... By the time I hit the towpath near Frazee house (about 28 miles or so) ALL I can do is walk. I ask Tanya Cady if she has any recommendations and she just says to keep walking and see what can be done at Station Road Bridge. OK, that is all I can do. I hobble on. I discover walking down the towpath that the only way the pain abates is if I turn my left foot in about 20-30 degrees (pigeon toed) and kind of walk a little sideways. It looks and feels awkward, and the next two miles elicits more "Are you OK?" questions than I could remember. **Fred Davis** catches me just before Station Bridge and I plead for his sage advice. He says all I can do is keep walking, and hope it goes away. Well, yeah, that is about it.

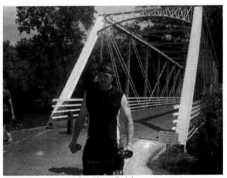

Station Bridge.

I come on in across the bridge, and tell Lasheda what is up, and she says, "What are you going to do? Drop out?" No. I have lots of time to rebound. I try a big glob of Icy Hot on the hip just under my shorts. It feels better for a few seconds, but that is not real.... just took my mind off it. Then it starts to get REALLY hot down there, oops, I globbed too much on, and my skin is probably very porous and receptive right now. And....OH GOD, I got some on the fedorkel!!!Oh oh oh! That does NOT feel good! I rush over to the bathroom and use a few handfuls of water from the sink to try to rinse off Willy. Damn that was uncomfortable! I will walk out of here and see what happens. I do just that. Josh and Texas Tony catch me around the Carriage Trail and we get to share most of that loop together, but when they run on a little longer than I can at one point, I let them go and keep walking. Right before the return to the towpath and turn back to Station Bridge there is a long downhill off of Carriage Trail. I resolve that I am going to run all the way down, no matter how much it hurts. I do, and it gets better. I am able to run about half of the distance back up the towpath on willpower. There is still pain, but it is either less, or I am ignoring it better.

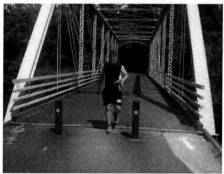

Station Bridge the second time in, actually feeling better...

I move fairly quickly through Station Bridge the second time, careful to avoid the Icy Hot. Josh got there and left, but Texas Tony is still there in a chair. It was his intention to take a short nap there he told us. I did try to change shoes into a pair of North Face trail shoes that I have, but after 10 steps they feel awkward so I switch right back to my faithful green gear. I did get new socks in the bargain though. I move on out of there, and in the next two miles run by Chippewa Creek which was one of the only sections of the course I had not seen, it is SO beautiful! I actually get tears for a while thinking of my brother I lost two summers ago and wondering how my Mom is. I check in each time I see Lasheda and she says she is fine...

I hit the aid station at Snowville Road (46.5) feeling a lot better and see Josh about to leave, and he says he wants to wait for me and run the next one together. Cool. We do...chit chatting the whole way (Harry Potter back on pause...) We both have run this section a good amount for the BT50k's and in training, so I generally know where we are the whole time.

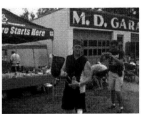

Boston Store. My great friend **Dimitrios** taking the following pictoral oddity...

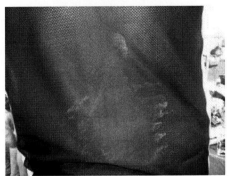

My sweat stains of salt on the back of my shirt demonstrated my **"can do attitude"** for the day! No idea how it formed like that, but it was funny.

Coming into Boston Store for the first time, I am feeling some potential hot spots on my soles so I elect to change socks and put duct tape over that area to protect it. It feels weird the first ten minutes or so out of Boston Store, but I soon forget it is there. This is not a great loop for me either. I am proud to have gone past 50 miles (my previous longest run) but I am gradually feeling worse and worse on that hip. I force myself to run the whole flat road prior to the long and steep hill towards Brandywine Falls. I am even still trying to run most flats and downhills on the far side of the Falls, but getting more and more frustrated because it is slow going, I know it, and it is hurting more and more to run. Maybe at this point I should have just walked for a few miles straight...I get back into Boston Store (56.5 miles)...losing time now. Over the 28 hour pace mark and close to 29. Dang. The next 4 miles is not easy and I know it ahead of time. Maybe this one moment it sucks to actually know the course, because I am dreading it. I get my lights...forget the waist light...just the Petzl and the light in the bottle expertly attached by Lasheda. Off I go.

I trudge through these trees, nearly brought to my knees by the struggle this eve. I do try running some of the flatter portions, I have to if I want to stay in this thing, but man it hurts. Hurts. The halfway point to Pine Lane is the end of the terrible 1/8th mile pine root infested lane right by the turnpike. It seems like it has taken me forever to get there, and I despair about my progress. I trudge.

And I trudge.

And I trudge.

I am almost surprised when I see the little Buckeye Trail map post that is 50 yards from the aid station. NOT because it was quick. Because I was in such a mental fog of just marching through the pain, that I really wasn't to aware of how far I had to go.... just on course, and keep moving.

The aid station brightens me a bit, because Lloyd is there, and so nice. Fred Davis is there! I thought perhaps he had dropped there due to a foot injury that I knew he had before the race, but I had somehow caught up to him! Wow! Hope renewed! Give me some good food, time to go? Guys how much ahead of cutoffs am I? 40 minutes according to Fred. One hour according to Lloyd. I figure Lloyd is being a good aid station captain and giving me hope, so I believe Fred and try my best to move faster out of there. The first two miles or so go well. Running the downs, the flats, climbing some hills at a walk. I hit the road. Things start to quickly HURT again! I run to specific obstacles to keep myself moving somewhat faster, but it hurts very badly each time. I walk to recover between and pick another goal and run. At some point the course hits Boston Mills Rd and then goes right onto a bike and hike path that I vaguely remember, but this portion is my lowest. Try as I might I can no longer run my little "goal" runs. The body hits that self-preservation boundary and I cannot push through it and will a run. I am sure perhaps I could run to save my life, but cannot pick it up for less right now.

I begin to despair. Really despair. I know I am losing time on the cutoff now. If I could run the last half of this five-mile section like I did the first, I would gain time, quite a bit of time. I can't. I hit the shorter section of woods on Boston Run Trail right before Happy Days aid station (65.7 miles) and I decide that at least I can give it everything I have to try to get credit for the whole 65.7. If I don't make the cutoff my official distance would be 60.8, I think. Kim comes back to find me in the edge of the woods and warn me of the dangerously close cutoff and I rally, but telling her that I am only trying to make the cutoff to get my first 100km+ run in the books.

I ran as hard as I could to that aid station tent, and they had everything ready to go, AND completed their job of getting me to leave there right at the cutoff.... Kim and I went maybe 1/8 mile up the way, and I stopped.... drinking some soup...I told Kim how sorry I was to let her down (although know she doesn't feel that way, I do...) but I can't pick up any time, I just could not move any faster. I had done it all, laid it all on the line to get there in the first place. I could handle going back home with the 65.7. I would NOT view this as a failure. I ran 16 miles further than ever before. I learned so much. I needed to be done this night. The next aid station was 3 miles, but unmanned, so the next place I could drop if I missed a cutoff, or decided to drop on my own, was 6 miles. I could not mentally commit to that 6-mile journey. I am sorry to Kim, and anyone who thinks I should have, but I am OK with it personally. I will be continuing to run hard, train hard. My next 100 miler will be Rocky Racoon in Texas in February, which is supposed to be less difficult than most. Then Mohican next summer, and back to BR. Before Rocky Raccoon, I will have Akron marathon (9-29), a planned Grand Canyon RimtoRimtoRim run - 50 miles (Oct. 13), The Slim Pickins FA 70miler, and probably 50k or 50miles at Art Moores FA in January. I won't dwell on it any longer than to say, don't worry about me, or my spirit, I have no regrets. I gave it 100% of what I had. *Besides, the book was just about over...what else was I going to listen to?*

I went home after we showed Kim the way to the 91.3 mile aid station so she could end up pacing Sean McCormack to his 9th 100 mile finish. He is the same guy I paced in at Mohican after Kim dropped at 76 miles. What a small world. We dropped off Texas Tony and a lady name Deb (I think) at the finish...I was really out of it at this point....foggy in the brain. 20 hours 42 minutes + on my feet. I went home, fell into bed, and awoke a few hours later, panicked I missed the finish of others, but it was only 730am. So I hobbled around to a shower.... got ready and we went to the finish line. Now it was raining. I had a little breakfast.... had just missed Josh finishing by a little. Actually got to see Kurt O. finish. I was so proud of him! And Tony the Tiger was there! An ultra marathoner to be sure! He has the scars to prove it. When he hit his usual distance at 26 miles, his body revolted and he went down hard on the trail. He literally says his head bounced off the dirt leaving behind some precious blood. His shoulder is also scraped up and a little on his legs.

The breakfast was delicious, even if I did feel a little suspect eating it for only running 65 miles. Thanks Bill! The awards ceremony was very, very nice, and I feel like it is my duty to watch it, even if I fall short. Those runners all deserve my admiration and respect for the journey they made. Kurt O. you are awesome! I know you won't even feel "average" for a while based on how much you suffered to get it done here. I hope the money you raised makes a HUGE difference for a child at the hospital.

Josh and **Michael Hayden** (2nd place finisher - 17 years old - also set a new record for 100 miles in the under 19 age group. 19:13 or so.) Mike stayed with us Sunday night and I took him to his flight home to Cali on Monday...he was a great guy. We recovered Monday morning by going to the pool, lifting a little, and running two miles on the track. He has a bright future ahead of him in running if he stays in it, and I think he will. The winner of the race was Mark Godale, a local running legend, in 16:07 I think.

I may post some more about my Mom at a later date. Right now it looks like she has lung cancer, but they did a biopsy on it today and will get results tomorrow morning, I will be there. I was supposed to be back at work today, but the combination of my soreness, and the worries about my Mom, are keeping me home another day or two. I have set up an appointment for Dr. Nilesh Shah (the local running doctor) for next week while home...I was hoping to get in today or tomorrow but could not. I will double check tomorrow in case he has a cancellation. I would really like to solve my hip issue, and of course, I think I know what is causing it, which will require a very minor surgery if I am right. We shall see.

I got to tell my goofy story while they were killing time before the awards. Somewhere around mile 22 or so, I am running, and over my Harry Potter I hear a huge CRACK! in the woods and turn to see a tree falling maybe 40 feet away...a big one. Wow! First time I have even seen a tree fall in person. For a minute I thought it was Kreacher the house elf apparating near me.... (Sorry, Harry Potter joke...you would have to read it.) Around 1.5 hours later, a little farther off trail 60-80 feet.... CRACK! Boom! A second tree falls! Weird. NEVER in my life...camping...in the army.... trail running...anything, had I ever seen a tree fall.... then two in less than two hours. hmmmm, Magic? Well if that wasn't, the race weekend sure was.

Chapter 8 – The wrap up

I believe I will wrap up this book with one last race report, my hometown marathon, the Road Runner Akron Marathon. I was battered, but not beaten from not finishing my first 100, but I always consider myself a person of perspective, and many people fail to finish their first 100. I ran further than I ever had before, and I will be back to finish this one and more next year. As the 100 memories began to fade, I turned my attention to training well for the Akron Marathon and shooting for that elusive sub 4 hour finish. I followed the training regimen in the book, and come race day, I truly felt ready.

SATURDAY, SEPTEMBER 29, 2007

Battling the Bird

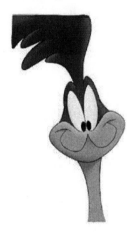

Tony and I went down and bopped around at the expo, enjoying seeing some running acquaintances. Tony picked up some very cool shades, and I nabbed a few of Chef Bill's pure fuel energy bars (soon to be available online, I think), as well as 4 packs of energy gels for the race from Vertical Runner. Also, I got a pair of running shorts I thought would work for the race. They are from Asics and have the compression shorts built right into them. I was skeptical to try something new on race day, but decided to risk it. If you remember the Cleveland marathon and my lovely green shorts, the chafing there was a nightmare. They only had a liner though, not full compression shorts. In case I forget to revisit it (I expect this to be a LONG blog post) the shorts were great! I want to get more of them now and will have to look around or online, for different colors. I got blue of course for the Akron Marathon.

I returned home and awaited the arrival of the Trail Goddess for the overnight prior to torturing her on the roads. Kim arrived from her stop at the expo and we chatted while I prepared a couple of batches of my pumpkin bread and muffins (yes Bill, from scratch.) As the first batch hit the ovens, we popped her new DVD about Massanutten into the player and started watching. It wasn't long before I was missing my ultra times and wondering if I would be off the weekend of Massanutten in 2008. I think I will focus my energy on finishing a more "entry level" 100 miler first.

Soon my wife was cooking the dinner and we were treated to very tasty spaghetti and salad. I tried to eat "just enough" to get my "carbo load" on, but not so much that I would be pooping it all out on race day. I completed some last minute prep actions prior to bedtime like printing out a pace band (**3:58 goal PACE**), trimming some stuff off of my shoes, printing some maps for my wife and kids to find me on race day, and even, yes, completing an artificially induced BM to lessen the chance of any race day surprises.

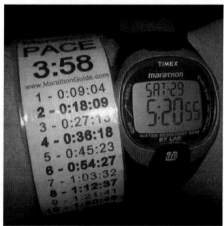

My crutch for the day - thank you www.marathonguide.com!

I got to sleep at a pretty decent hour for me and slept right through the night. Alarms went off at 4 am and I arose (as did Kim) and went to the kitchen to get some calories in 3 hours before the race as recommended. I drank a chocolate Slimfast, ate one packet of sugar free oatmeal, and had a pumpkin muffin. I would not drink anything else pre-race hoping to keep urination delays to a minimum.

Kim spent the morning in the kitchen telling me about a dream she had where she was at an ultra and there was a lake that had Godzilla in it, with all kinds of drama surrounding this issue. Hmmmm... a monster eh? I had a monster to slay today, my 4-hour nemesis.

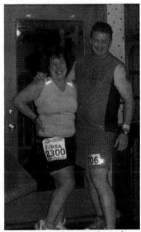
5:20 a.m. getting ready to leave!

We left for the race at 5:40 am, knowing we would have to sit awhile in the car, but we had plenty to chat about. After a bit though, we wanted to search out fellow runners and left the car for the start line. I left behind my jacket, because a close friend gave it to me, and I didn't want to ditch it at the start. Enroute to the start I ran into Dr. Joe Salwan and Bob Clark along with the rest of their relay team. We continued up to the starting line tent and I was pretty chilly just wearing a sleeveless mesh-like t-shirt. Inside the tent I found I could stay a touch warmer by standing right under some exposed incandescent bulbs. They had plenty of clothing donation bins and I should have brought an older t-shirt to wear and ditch just prior to start.

I would run into the Inca Princess in the potty line while waiting to

153

take my last minute pee, and also see Maria in street clothes and looking good (she has an injury right now precluding running a bit longer.) Chef Bill and I would find one another, we were both running with the 4:00 pace group and had agreed to more or less ignore each other verbally to avoid wasting energy talking. Kurt popped up and said hi in the starting corral. A few minutes prior to start Tony found me and gave me a fist pump wishing me luck. He has been such a huge inspiration and help to me getting ready for this. I imagine Tony will **always** be my marathon mentor in my mind. He had to then move up to the very front of the corral for the start. Tony was shooting for a 2:55 today.

I tried to figure out why there was a pace sign on the side of the corral for 3:56 or 9:00 per mile pace, but yet our pace group was for 4:00 finish (or 9:10 per mile pace.) I lined up with our Pace team leader Dave, but didn't say much, because as mentioned before, I wanted to be quiet while running. A minute or so before the start Dave offered his throwaway jacket to anyone cold, and after no one took it, I grabbed it and wore it for like 90 seconds before heaving it off to the side. I didn't want to run with a jacket on. Off we go, and I started my stopwatch as I crossed the starting line, some 1:30 or so after the official start. This would help me to see my actual time as my chip would be recording it.

As we finished the first mile and were almost off the Y Bridge going north, the leaders started to come back down the other side. I looked hard for Tony, but only ended up seeing Vince in the lead pack before giving up and focusing on my race. I was dismayed at first not to see Tony very close to the front until I remembered that the half marathon runners were in there blazing a fast track. Looping back for our southbound leg across the Y Bridge. We were still all bottled up at this point, but things were ever so gradually starting to thin out.

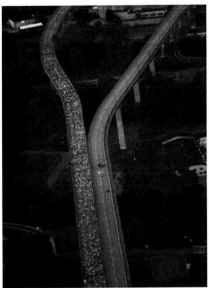

Mile 1 - crossing the Y bridge (from the Akron Beacon Journal, Paul Tople)
Any questions why locals call it the "Y" bridge anymore? It is actually the All America Bridge.

Back through town, and head south, I felt it coming. By the 4-mile mark and rest stop there would be no option. Next port-o-john and I had a date, and *I couldn't stand her up* (umm, literally folks.) I was lucky though, and had almost zero wait for a open john. I really felt like so much came out, I was going to be good all day now. Dang! I thought I took care of this the night before. Well, I would just come out and catch the 4-hour group as gradually as possible to save energy.

One half mile later on the sidewalk, I see a prone dead body.... just lying there. I was kind of shocked. Who knows how that cat died?

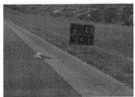

(I didn't carry my camera; I found this on Google....)

Onward we go...I see the pace group and I am ever so slightly gathering them up. By mile 5.5 or so, I am back with Bill and the group. By mile 6, I am headed for the next port-o-john, but this time I only have to pee. Not an option though, I HAVE to pee. Damn. I have to wait a little for a potty this time, which sucked. I probably stood there for a full minute or so.

OK, WHEW! Feel better now, get back out and start reeling them back in again. I do it again in about a mile and half, using the downhills to gain ground with less effort. Mile 8.5 or so comes, and, yes, you guessed it, I have to pee again. WTF over? So I peel away from Bill, by now he is wondering what is going on with me. I get to the potties and have to wait again...this time the wait is bothering me and taking too long...I was thinking about moving over and going on the abandoned building, when finally one opens up and I dash in, pee, and get out.
OK, please now, let's just run the rest of the day, OK body?

Up Brown Street and onto the University of Akron campus, the end of my second loop is near and I am happy to have the towpath ahead of me, and the long downhill to get to it. I know as I turn left in front of the Y bridge that I have another stop though. This is getting crazy! This time is going to be full service like the first stop. I open up my stride and make some distance on my pace group going down the Howard Street hill, and get to the two potties at the start of the towpath. I wait, and wait, and wait, and get in and try to hurry. The seat has stuff all over it (some of which was vomit) and I HAVE to clean that off, and then do my best again to be thorough but quick. Again, I am sure leaving that this is my last stop of this type. (If this were a big ultra I would be pulled from the race for weight loss!)

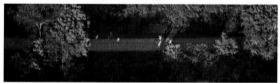

The towpath (miles 11-15+) (Photo via the Akron Beacon Journal, Paul Tople)

The towpath was wonderful and relatively soft compared to the last 11 miles. I don't see the pace group all the way down the towpath, but do reel in Kurt O. again. He had caught me briefly on the streets and "tagged" me with a little disc he gives people while running to solicit donations for the Children's Hospital. As a rule, I ignore these kinds of solicitations, but Kurt really cares about this effort and I respect him, so I think I will cave in and donate. So, I caught him and passed him with no fanfare, figuring I might see him again, especially if I have to poop again! When I ran past the 15-mile mark near the end of the towpath my head was swiveling around looking for where Tony hides his Gatorade in a tree. I didn't see any likely candidates.

Off the towpath there is a short uphill to get to Sand Run Park, which I am also looking forward to. There is a lot of commotion with relay teams handing off at the start of Sand Run, and I enjoyed passing this area with all the people. Now I know I am getting deep into my last big loop of the race, but I am also fighting to catch the pace group and hoping my excretionary excursions are at an end. I am feeling a little sore now, but I have been there before and will just ignore it. After a mile or more into Sand Run there is a stream that crosses the road. In a trail race we would laugh at that and run right through, but roadrunners have none of that and there was a temporary bridge in place that allowed us to cross the water with dry feet. (I think running through the stream would give this marathon character - although it needs nothing else, it was a GREAT, fun, well-organized race in my opinion.)

The stream is the low point and then you start uphill. Mile 17 comes and I check my time, just about 30 seconds off my pace band of 3:58 pace, and I promptly find a tree and go pee...no waiting this time, just the peeing. That makes 5 bathroom stops if you are counting!

I keep going, and this section is a long uphill on which I do my best at maintaining pace. I am thinking about the joy of making my goal. I am thinking how temporary my discomfort is...all kinds of things to keep me going at pace. I turn the left onto Revere Rd and I know I am at the far point now of my large loop! Keep going Mike! I see my neighbors standing right near this corner and give a hello, one of the few words I utter all race long. I think the only other things I said were when Bill pointed out I was going too fast early on, I told him I was building time for a poop, and when I saw my girls just before the finish line I hollered out my love.

Somewhere going down Revere Rd, I have a funny sensation in my right leg. No pain, but I have this feeling like my leg could buckle if I try to go to hard. I was thinking that the muscles were just fatigued and I just tried to stay right below the threshold of that feeling. It didn't really make me go slower; it was just something I noticed. It would come and go over the next 4 miles until I got on the final stretch. I was relieved to get to Market Street and see a long flat stretch of road. Turning off of Market I am anticipating Debi's house and party in a few minutes, but also noticing that I am almost 5 minutes behind when I said I would get there, or 3 minutes behind the 4-hour pace now. I really do my best and as I get to Debi's I am looking for my girls, I haven't seen them yet during the race. No girls, but I do get a HUGE lift when I see the signs for all of us in Debi's front yard. Many of our running group had signs and mine simply said "Mike K" with two jets in silhouette below the words. I was smiling for a full 2-3 minutes from that. Thank you Debi! That was so cool.

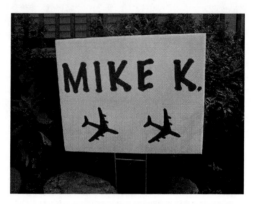

As my smile faded, flowing tears replaced it. Yes, I cried and I don't mind admitting it. I had put a song on my mp3 player, which always gets to me. It is called "Wild Mountain Thyme" and was the song we all sang at my brother's funeral. I was happily crying remembering my brother, but at the same time thinking that onlookers must think I have a bad injury or something. Sure, I felt like crap, but the tears were for John.

The tears just seemed to morph into a strange resolve that the mountain ahead of me, Mount Garman, would not claim me. I saw it looming, and everything within me said to just walk it briskly and run from the top, but my resolve built and I said NO! I will run it! I did and when I crested the top I was so relieved to feel that my climbing was more or less done. I had to now start building back some time to try to recapture 4 hours. Dash in to Stan Hywet Hall's grounds and back out, and now I have the mostly flat section out to Market Street. I keep my resolve up to give all I got and pass a bunch of people heading out to Market. I am thinking about when I ran through here with Bill Bailey on the Indian run in April and now I am just a few minutes behind him. Thankfully now, all my peeing and pooping is behind me, but I fear I don't have enough real estate to make up my deficit.

I open up whatever I have left, remembering that Tony says the bad feelings are mostly in my head. I am thinking "Go Mike Go!" I pass a few people going down Market. I am acutely aware when people pass me of whether they are marathon runners or relay runners. I am not supposed to be racing them, but it does make me feel better when the people passing me are mostly relay team members, having only run a 6 mile or so leg.

I know when I hit the 25-mile mark with something like 8 minutes or so left that 4 hours has slipped my grip. My proverbial "monster" will live to fight me another day, same as Kim's Godzilla dreams. But I have a mile left, and my spirit is not done, even if 4 hours has gone away. I crank up my pace to whatever I have left, and I think I ran the last mile in about 8:20 or so, determined to get my PR as low as possible. The **last mile** though, was from 25.2 to 26.2, and that two tenths was too much to let me get in less than 4 hours.

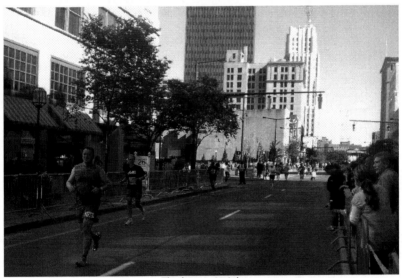

The home stretch

I see the girls, turn down into the stadium, and do my best on the warning track to the line. I crossed the line in 4:02:48, an overall pace of 9:16 per mile. A new PR by almost 10 minutes. Tony is there right after, and I relay my disappointment and apologies, but he is proud of

159

me, and will not hear it. I get a big hug from Tony and gather my goodies, the medal, and the Mylar blanket making me feel like a rock star. In true fashion, I profusely thank the volunteers I see for being there. One sweet old lady bends down and clips my time chip off of my shoe, making me smirk that she can now bend down better than I can.

Up to the concessions level and I am re-hydrating and grabbing a couple food bags. I sweet-talked the volunteer into two of them. I ate the turkey and cheese off of the sandwiches and one of the energy bars. I am moving slow but find my family soon, and we choose to waste little time and get going. I just want to sit down and shower at this point.

I look back on the race and it is hard when I realize the bathroom breaks took me over 4 hours (suggestions anyone? Imodium or something?) If I could have ran through without stopping I would have been under 4 for sure. Bill Bailey did 3:57:47 with only one stop to pee. Tony fell a touch shy of the 2:55 hitting 2:59:10, but you know... he IS old, so what are you going to do. One of the funniest realizations I had this week is that while Tony gets older, and I get fitter and faster, there MAY come a day when our marathon times converge and we can run a race together! I am quite sure that day is still far off though.

No cats were harmed in the making of this blog post. The cat was already dead and I merely documented it's passing. I may have a supplemental post regarding the marathon when pictures come in from Maria. Don't forget to watch for blog posts from Red, Bill Bailey, Kim, and Maria regarding the race!

If you made it this far, I thank you for caring enough about my story to keep reading. I know now at this point in my life that I can never go back to who I was becoming before and expect to be happy. There must be adventure, and there must be fun.

In the next year, I plan on trying at least three 100-mile races, many repeat marathons, and a few new ones. I want to run across the state of Ohio (over 5 days probably.) I want to mix in some long bike rides, and some good swims too. 4 hours will fall in the marathon.

There is this idea I have had many times while trying to put into words what I have gone through in the last year and a half; I will try once more. If you are in a situation in your life like I was, and you want to make a change, you CAN! This is the kicker though, do it because you want to, not because someone else thinks you should, or you think you are supposed to, or some external reason. Find what you want and go get it! It is there for the taking. In the end, you will **not** be a better person if you lose weight or get in shape, your value to the world and those around you lies in your actions and emotions, and not your waste size; that being said, you just might find that you are a happier person, and there is nothing wrong with that.

As of the writing of this book, I keep my blog at www.fitfromfat.blogspot.com and there are many side adventures that never made it to this book, but are in the archives, and there will be many future adventures to come.

Thank you!